The Complete Paleo Cookbook for Beginners

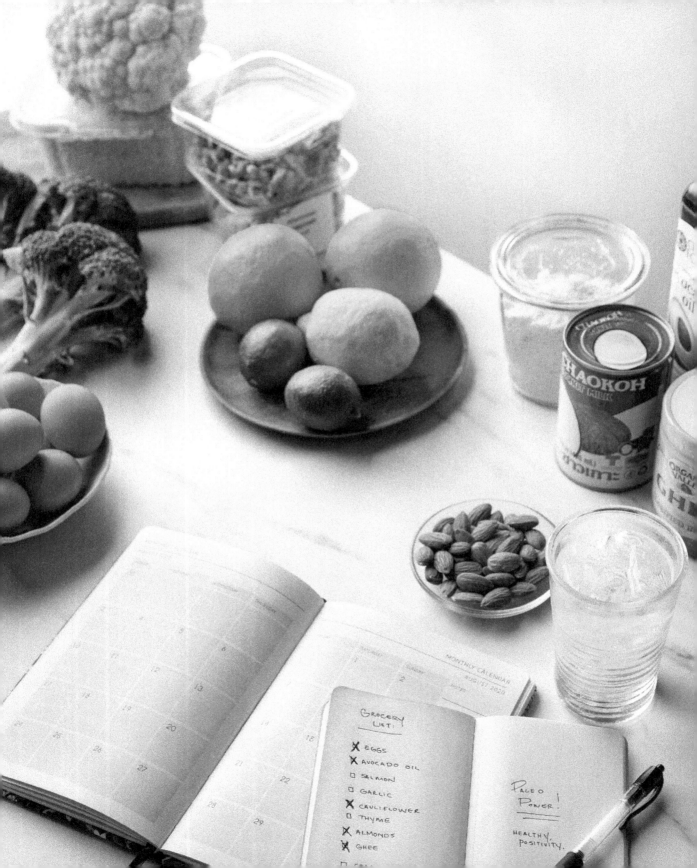

GROCERY
LIST:

☒ EGGS
☒ AVOCADO OIL
☐ SALMON
☐ GARLIC
☒ CAULIFLOWER
☐ THYME
☒ ALMONDS
☒ GHEE

PALEO
POWER!

HEALTHY
POSITIVITY.

The Complete PALEO Cookbook for Beginners

Recipes and Meal Plans for
Weight Loss and Better Health

Kinsey Jackson, MS, CNS®
Sally Johnson, MA, RD

ROCKRIDGE
PRESS

For general information on our other products and services or to obtain technical support, please contact our Customer Care Department within the United States at (866) 744-2665, or outside the United States at (510) 253-0500.

Rockridge Press publishes its books in a variety of electronic and print formats. Some content that appears in print may not be available in electronic books, and vice versa.

TRADEMARKS: Rockridge Press and the Rockridge Press logo are trademarks or registered trademarks of Callisto Media Inc. and/or its affiliates, in the United States and other countries, and may not be used without written permission. All other trademarks are the property of their respective owners. Rockridge Press is not associated with any product or vendor mentioned in this book.

Interior and Cover Designer: Stephanie Sumulong
Art Producer: Maya Melenchuk
Editor: Kelly Koester
Production Manager: Martin Worthington
Production Editor: Melissa Edeburn

Photography © Evi Abeler, p. 51; © Shannon Douglas, p. 89; © 2021 Hélène DuJardin, cover and pp. 49, 80, 99, 100, 102, 113, 123, 124, 133, 135, 144; © Shea Evans, p. 167; © Nadine Greeff, pp. x, 158; © Biz Jones, p. 65; © Darren Muir, pp. vi, 44, 63, 79, 169; © Andrew Purcell, p. 19; © Marija Vidal, p. 121; © Elysa Weitala, pp. ii, 20, 59, 60, 69, 91, 107, 117, 139, 147, 157, 170.

Food styling by Anna Hampton, cover and pp. 49, 80, 99, 100, 102, 113, 124, 133, 135, 144.

Author photo of Kinsey Jackson courtesy of Naomi D. Sheikin. Photography Author photo of Sally Johnson courtesy of Denise Morris Photography.

Paperback ISBN: 978-1-63878-461-6
eBook ISBN: 978-1-63878-764-8
R0

This book is dedicated to you, dear reader.
We commend you for having the strength and
courage to take your health into your own hands.
By doing so, you are truly making this a healthier
and more sustainable world to live in.
A new you is only a few short weeks away. Enjoy!

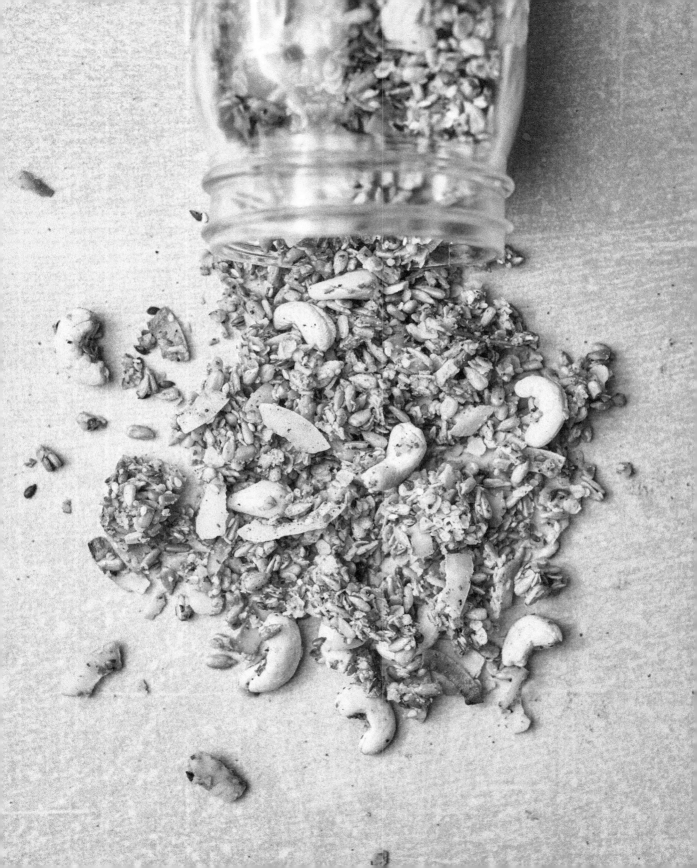

Contents

Introduction

Welcome to *The Complete Paleo Cookbook for Beginners*, your guide to feeling your absolute best simply by eating the foods that nature intended. Perhaps you've heard a remarkable Paleo success story about profound weight loss or the reversal of chronic disease. Or maybe you're just curious or looking to try something new. Whatever your motivation, this book will have you up and running with the Paleo diet in no time.

As Paleo nutritionists, we've witnessed countless individuals achieve dramatic and life-changing results, and on a personal level, we've both experienced how transformative eating Paleo can be.

After following a vegetarian diet for nearly 25 years, Kinsey was diagnosed with multiple autoimmune diseases, including rheumatoid arthritis, lupus, hypothyroidism, and alopecia. By transitioning from vegetarian to Paleo, she used food as her medicine to reverse her autoimmunity and keep it in remission.

By rejecting the standard dietary advice and adopting a Paleo diet and lifestyle, Sally lost unwanted pounds that had been creeping on over the years and resolved two decades of IBS, GERD, gingivitis bordering on periodontitis, and other debilitating inflammatory conditions.

We know firsthand the power of Paleo, and we can't wait for you to experience it, too.

Many people fail to realize that their health issues are intimately connected to the foods they eat. Obesity, heart disease, diabetes, dementia, cancers, mood disorders, allergies, body pain, headaches, infertility, and skin problems (to name a few) all have something in common . . . and that something is *inflammation*. The presence of *chronic* inflammation underlies many illnesses and can trigger the expression of diseases to which we are genetically predisposed (autoimmune disease, for example, runs in families). However, genetic predisposition does *not* mean destiny. In fact, we have the power to turn off genes that are causing disease simply by shutting down the production of inflammation in our bodies. And it all starts with diet.

By following the meal plans in this book, you'll quickly realize that Paleo is far from yet another boring, bland, restrictive diet. On the contrary—the meals are delicious, easy to prepare, and extremely satisfying. Many take fewer than 30 minutes to make, contain fewer than five ingredients, or require only a single vessel for cooking!

By the end of chapter 1, you'll understand why your body was designed to eat Paleo. Chapter 2 is your quick-start guide. The remainder of the book contains 85 recipes that will keep you eating Paleo for months after you conquer the two-week meal plans.

We're so excited for you to discover how amazing it feels to fuel your body with nourishing, delicious Paleo foods. Are you ready? A new and improved you is only a few weeks away!

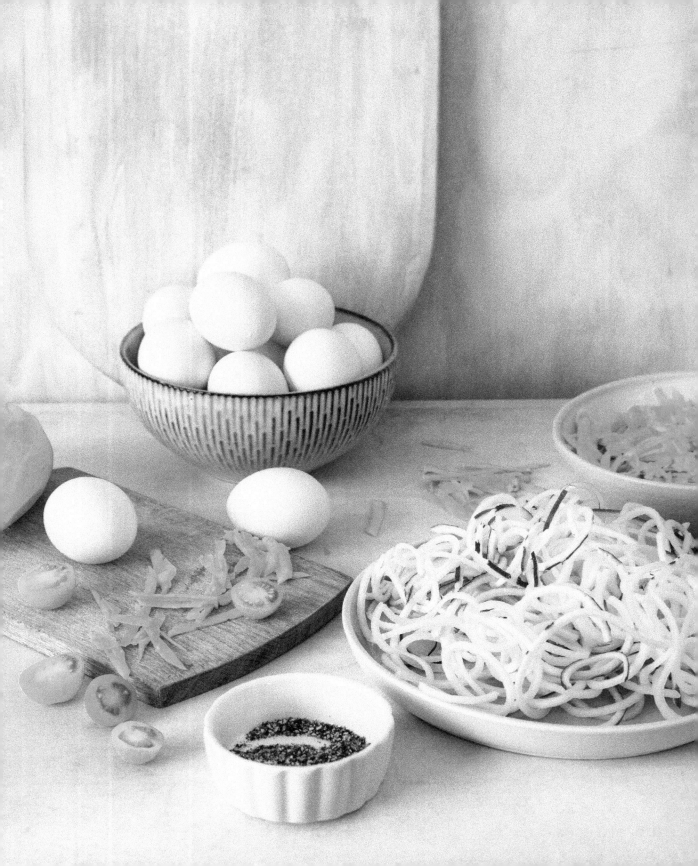

CHAPTER 1

Paleo 101

Welcome to Paleo! If your goal is to lose weight, reverse chronic disease, or look and feel your absolute best, then you're in the right place. The Paleo diet is your key to achieving optimal health. This chapter walks you through the foods you'll be eating and avoiding, the tools you'll need to make the diet work, and the steps you'll take to make the transition as seamless as possible. You'll be a Paleo pro in no time at all!

So You Want to Go Paleo

The Paleo (short for Paleolithic) diet is modeled on humankind's original diet, the way humans have eaten for the vast majority of the time that we have inhabited this Earth. When we eat the way nature intended, our bodies heal from the inside out. In recent generations, our perception of "normal" eating has been greatly skewed. The introduction of fast food, processed foods, refined grains, and vegetable oils is largely to blame for the current epidemics of obesity and chronic disease. Remove these foods from your diet, and you'll quickly see that your body was not designed to process them.

Most of us believe that aging inevitably equates to declining health and ability. But eating a proper diet is one of the best ways we can help ourselves "age gracefully." The Paleo diet combats inflammation, which begins in the gut. The majority of modern diseases are rooted in inflammation. Even Hippocrates recognized this fact over 2,000 years ago when he wrote, "All disease begins in the gut." Obesity, autoimmunity, diabetes, allergies, cardiovascular disease, depression, anxiety, and countless other disorders can be triggered by excess inflammation in your body. Reduce inflammation, and many of these conditions naturally go into remission. Researchers are recognizing that when we heal the gut, the production of inflammation ceases and overall health improves.

A Paleo Primer

Let's dive into what Paleo is and why it works. The Paleo diet mimics the types of foods humans ate prior to the Agricultural Revolution (a mere 10,000 years or 400 generations ago). These foods include meat, seafood, eggs, fresh vegetables, fruits, nuts, and seeds. Paleo foods are chock-full of vitamins and minerals, antioxidants, fiber, beneficial fatty acids, and low-glycemic carbohydrates that promote good health. The Paleo diet does not contain refined sugars or grains, beans, dairy, unhealthy fats, or processed foods, which are often the cause of weight gain and many other health problems.

REAL, UNPROCESSED FOOD

At its core, Paleo is a real-food diet composed of whole, unprocessed ingredients as close to their natural form as possible. Processed foods—like those found in packages with long shelf lives—are almost always unhealthy. If a food can be stored for months or years before its expiration, it's likely that chemicals have been added to preserve its longevity. Because our bodies do not know how to process these additives, they get stored away in our body fat, where they can continue to wreak havoc on our health for years to come.

Processed foods and fast food are also devoid of the vitamins and minerals your body needs to function optimally and remain disease-free. Although some processed foods are fortified with vitamins, these nutrients are often in a form that is difficult for the body to utilize. Paleo foods, on the other hand, contain vitamins and minerals that are bioavailable, meaning they are in a form that is readily recognized and utilized by the human body.

NUTRITIONAL DENSITY AND SATISFACTION

Consuming real, nutrient-dense foods is one key to a long and healthy life. Nutrient-dense foods give you the most bang for your buck; you need to consume less of them to feel full and meet your nutritional requirements.

Paleo takes things a step further by removing foods that were introduced as a result of the Agricultural Revolution, including all grains and legumes (beans). Grains and legumes contain chemicals called antinutrients that are irritating to the gut lining and trigger the production of inflammation through a process known as leaky gut syndrome.

BALANCED MEALS

All foods break down into the three macronutrients: carbohydrates, proteins, and fats. Our bodies convert these macronutrients into energy, which is used for healing and growth. The ratio of these macronutrients in your diet is known as the macronutrient ratio. Although other diets may contain an approximate macronutrient ratio of 50 percent carbohydrates, 15 percent protein, and 35 percent fat, the macronutrient ratio of a Paleo diet is roughly 20 percent carbohydrates, 25 percent protein, and 55 percent fat. Our Paleolithic ancestors consumed far fewer carbohydrates and more fat than modern humans do today. By increasing your dietary fat intake, your body learns how to burn it for fuel (this is known as becoming "fat-adapted" or "keto-adapted") and can also start utilizing stored body fat for energy.

For any given Paleo meal, at least half of your plate will be filled with plant foods, and the remainder with animal foods. This provides your body with readily available fiber, macronutrients and micronutrients, amino acids, and the healthy fats it needs to heal from the inside out.

TOP BENEFITS OF EATING PALEO

Numerous benefits—among them weight loss, increased energy, reduced inflammation, balanced blood sugar, fewer aches and pains, fewer allergy symptoms, clearer skin, enhanced immunity, and improved mood—result from feeding your body the foods it was designed to eat.

Weight loss is a well-known benefit of the Paleo diet related to the lower carbohydrate and higher fat content of Paleo foods. When you become less carbohydrate dependent and begin utilizing more fat for fuel, your body can finally burn off that extra stored fat tissue. In addition, much of the excess weight people carry around is due to inflammation. You'll quickly witness the anti-inflammatory nature of Paleo as you lose pounds of inflammation, which also radically reduces your risk for cardiovascular disease and other chronic diseases.

Improved energy is another wonderful benefit of eating Paleo. A large percentage of our energy goes to replacing the gut lining every few days. When you make the switch to eating gut-healing Paleo foods, this energy is liberated for use by other parts of your body, which translates to increased energy for you!

Better digestion results when we remove processed foods from our diet. The fiber found in all the wonderful vegetables and fruits you'll be enjoying facilitates better elimination and reduced digestive symptoms while helping populate the beneficial bacteria in your gut. Healthy gut flora are critical for good digestion, overall health, and wellness.

Improvement of health conditions ranging from the aches and pains of aging to cardiovascular disease, diabetes, autoimmunity, and other chronic health disorders takes place when eating a real-food diet. By avoiding non-Paleo foods, you are reducing inflammation and balancing your blood sugars, and greatly reducing your risk for many chronic diseases in the process. Many people experience a complete reversal of health issues within only a few months of transitioning to a Paleo diet.

PALEO FAQ

As you dive into Paleo, you'll likely have questions about how to customize the diet for your unique needs. Here are the top five questions we hear from Paleo newbies.

I have a lot of weight to lose. Should I be doing keto or a low-carb diet instead? Although the keto diet has become popular for rapid weight loss, it is not a sustainable diet for many people in the long term and can lead to health issues when followed incorrectly. Paleo, which is also a low-carb diet, allows more carbs than keto but will yield the weight loss you desire. If you have a lot of weight to lose, consider moderating your carbohydrate intake more strictly.

I need to gain weight. Will this diet work for me? If you need to gain weight or if you exercise heavily, are elderly, or are cooking for a growing child, you will likely need to include more carbohydrates in the form of starchy vegetables, fruits, nuts, and seeds (smoothies and liquid meals work, too).

I have a chronic disease (like autoimmune disease or diabetes). Will Paleo help? Paleo can do wonders for reversing many chronic diseases. If you have diabetes, you may need to be stricter with carbohydrate intake and minimize your intake of starchy vegetables, fruits, and Paleo sweeteners. Many people with autoimmune conditions feel great eating strictly Paleo, whereas others need to take things a step further by following the autoimmune protocol (AIP), which also removes eggs, nightshade vegetables, nuts, seeds, alcohol, and other potential trigger foods. As always, everyone has different needs—be sure to consult your healthcare professional before embarking on any new diet.

I like to eat at restaurants. Is this diet doable when eating out? Eating Paleo at restaurants is quite easy! Let your server know about your food restrictions up front. You'll want to order dishes that contain only meat and vegetables. Salads are a great option, but ask for olive oil and vinegar as a dressing (or bring your own).

continued →

continued

I don't have any digestive symptoms when I eat dairy, grains, and beans. Why do I have to give them up? More often than not, the foods to which your body is intolerant do *not* give you digestion issues. Rather, they can cause a host of symptoms ranging from headaches to sleep disorders, fatigue, skin conditions, weight gain, inflammation, and chronic diseases that we may not attribute to diet. The gold standard for identifying hidden food allergies is an elimination diet, where you avoid questionable foods for up to six weeks, then gradually reintroduce them, monitoring yourself for symptoms as they are reintroduced. Grains and beans are big culprits, causing leaky gut in nearly every person who consumes them. Up to 70 percent of the population has some degree of dairy intolerance. For these reasons, it is wise to remove these foods from your diet to assess how you actually tolerate them.

Foods to Avoid, Eat in Moderation, and Embrace

For hundreds of thousands of years, humans ate a Paleo diet. Only in recent history have we diverged from this way of eating and incorporated foods that strain our digestion and put a toxic load on our detox organs. Now that you know why you want to eat Paleo, let's dive into the nitty-gritty details of how to do it: which foods to avoid, enjoy, or eat in moderation.

AVOID THESE FOODS COMPLETELY

Paleo excludes certain foods for a good reason: they're known dietary disruptors that contribute to weight gain, inflammation, and disease. The following foods—and any foods that contain these as ingredients—are to be strictly avoided on the Paleo diet.

All grains such as gluten-free grains, wheat, rice, corn, quinoa, oats, and cereal.

All beans (legumes) such as pinto beans, black beans, lentils, chickpeas, soybeans, and peanuts.

All dairy such as milk, cheese, yogurt, whey, and other dairy-derived products.

All vegetable oils such as canola, corn, soy, peanut, sunflower, safflower, and other heavily processed oils.

All processed foods especially when the label includes the words "artificial," "refined," or "hydrogenated."

All artificial sweeteners such as sucralose (Splenda), aspartame (Equal, NutraSweet), acesulfame-K (Sweet One), white stevia (Truvia), and saccharin (Sweet'N Low).

Most types of sugar such as agave, cane sugar or syrup, white and brown sugar, brown rice syrup, high-fructose corn syrup, and anything ending in -ose (soda, sweetened beverages, and fruit juices also fall under this category).

EAT THESE FOODS IN MODERATION

The following foods should be eaten only in moderation, especially if you want to lose weight, are struggling with a chronic disease, or need to regulate your blood sugar levels.

Starchy vegetables such as potatoes, sweet potatoes, and other tubers are concentrated in carbohydrates, which can spike blood sugar levels and make weight loss difficult.

Fruits such as apples, grapes, oranges, and melons contain nutrients and antioxidants, but beware of their carbohydrate content. Fruit should be limited to two pieces per day or less. Fruit juices and all types of liquid carbohydrates should be avoided altogether. Eat fruit with a protein and/or fat, such as nut butter, to reduce its blood sugar impact.

Nuts and seeds should be limited to a small handful a day or less. Also use nut and seed flours, butters, and milks in moderation. Eat a variety of different nut types to prevent developing intolerance to any one variety. Read ingredient labels to ensure that nuts, seeds, and products derived from them contain no added oils or sugars.

Dark chocolate (at least 70% to 85% cacao) is allowed in moderation. Be sure to read the labels to ensure that all the ingredients are Paleo-friendly.

Alcohol that is made from fermented fruits or vegetables (e.g., wine, tequila, potato vodka, gin, etc.) is allowed on the Paleo diet, up to two servings per day. Steer clear of beer, which is made from grains. Be mindful that alcohol can derail your efforts at weight loss and overcoming disease.

Caffeine, including coffee, is allowed in moderation (up to two cups per day). Use only Paleo-friendly creamers like almond or coconut milk, with no added sweeteners.

ENJOY THESE FOODS FREELY

The following foods can be enjoyed freely on the Paleo diet. When possible, select organic plant foods, wild-caught fish and shellfish, and grass-fed, pasture-raised meats. Opt for organic, cold-pressed, unrefined oils, and animal fats from pasture-raised animals. These foods contain the highest levels of nutrition while minimizing toxins. If you can't afford these higher-end options, however, it's certainly not a Paleo deal breaker.

All types of meats such as beef, poultry, pork, lamb, game, and organ meats.

All types of seafood, including fish and shellfish.

All types of nonstarchy vegetables such as dark leafy greens and sea vegetables.

Low-glycemic fruits such as avocados, limes, lemons, and berries.

Eggs from any type of animal.

Herbs and spices, including unrefined natural salt.

Healthy fats such as coconut oil, coconut cream, and full-fat coconut milk; extra-virgin olive oil, avocado oil, and macadamia nut oil; and grass-fed ghee, tallow, lard, and other animal fats.

ARE THESE PALEO-FRIENDLY?

Here's a rundown on the Paleo-friendliness of some frequently debated foods and drinks.

Butter and ghee are dairy products, but they are allowed on the Paleo diet, especially when they come from grass-fed animals. They are well tolerated by most and offer tremendous health benefits—ghee even more so than regular butter, because it is pure butterfat with the allergenic carbohydrate and protein portions removed.

Green beans and peas are the exception to the no-legume rule. In their green state, these legumes contain very few gut-irritating antinutrients (compared to dried legumes) and are safe to consume in moderation.

Natural sweeteners such as raw honey, maple syrup, molasses, and coconut sugar can be consumed in moderation. Still, these sources of sugar can interfere with weight loss and healing, so they are best kept to a minimum.

Potatoes are a nightshade vegetable and are technically Paleo. Because they are a concentrated source of starchy carbohydrates, they should be avoided or kept to a minimum for those with a lot of weight to lose, blood sugar disorders, or autoimmunity.

Processed meats like bacon and deli meats are allowed on the Paleo diet if they do not contain preservatives and their only ingredients are meat, salt, and herbs.

Salt gets a bad reputation, but it is essential for life and health. You can use salt liberally in your Paleo cooking. Just opt for a natural, unrefined salt like sea salt and avoid common table salt, which contains preservatives and other unhealthy additives.

Quinoa is classified as a pseudograin. Although technically a seed, it has grainlike characteristics. Because it contains gut-irritating antinutrients, it is not allowed on the Paleo diet, along with other pseudograins, such as buckwheat and amaranth.

FOODS TO ENJOY, MODERATE, OR AVOID ON THE PALEO DIET

FOODS TO ENJOY FREELY	FOODS TO EAT IN MODERATION	FOODS TO AVOID COMPLETELY
All types of meat and eggs	High-quality deli meats, bacon, and other processed meats	Processed meats containing chemical additives
All types of wild seafood	Farmed seafood	Seafood containing high levels of mercury that appears on the EWG's Consumer Guide to Seafood (see page 172)
All types of nonstarchy vegetables	Starchy vegetables	Conventionally raised produce that appears on the EWG's Dirty Dozen list
Low-glycemic fruits such as avocados, limes, lemons, and berries	Other fruits	Fruit juices and other sugary drinks
Coconut products: coconut cream, full-fat coconut milk	Nut and seed milks	Dairy products
Healthy plant oils: coconut, avocado, and olive	Nut and some seed oils: walnut, macadamia, sesame, flax, and pumpkin	Unhealthy plant oils: vegetable, canola, sunflower, safflower, corn, soy, peanut, and grapeseed
Pasture-raised or organic animal fats: lard, tallow, schmaltz, grass-fed ghee and butter (if tolerated), and others	Fats from conventionally raised animals	Artificial trans fats
Organic herbs, spices, and natural, unrefined salt	Conventionally raised herbs and spices	Common table salt
Paleo-friendly foods in nontoxic packaging: coconut milk, tomatoes, olives, bone broth, protein bars, etc.	Minimally processed foods: nuts and seeds, nut/seed/tuber flours and butters, and canned foods	Foods that are highly processed, refined, hydrogenated, or made from artificial ingredients; all grains and their derivatives; peanuts and peanut butter
Water and herbal teas	Caffeine, coffee, and alcohol derived from non-grain sources	Coffee alternatives and alcohol derived from grains
	Green beans, green peas, snow peas, and snap peas	All beans and legumes
	Dark chocolate and natural sweeteners	Sugar and artificial sweeteners

PALEO LIKE A PRO

1. **Prep ahead.** Meal prepping involves assembling part or all of your meal(s) in advance to minimize the work required at mealtime. This could involve washing, chopping, and storing veggies in containers, cooking and refrigerating or freezing meats, or assembling everything in the slow cooker the night before. It's helpful to choose two days per week to do some meal preparation.

2. **Cook in bulk.** Batch cooking involves making large amounts of food at once—either lots of different meals or a large amount of one thing (like bone broth, snacks, hard-boiled eggs, and soups). You can then freeze or refrigerate these foods so they're quick to grab for future use. When batch cooking and meal prepping, be sure to label and date everything to avoid confusion later.

3. **Dinner for breakfast.** One of the easiest ways to save time on Paleo is to utilize leftovers, such as having leftover dinner for breakfast or lunch the next day. Many of us are accustomed to eating carb-rich foods like cereal and baked goods for breakfast. Starting your day with healthy fats and proteins instead is an easy-to-digest way to break your fast.

4. **Time-saving tools.** A few kitchen tools can seriously expedite your food preparation. Instead of chopping, grating, mixing, and slicing by hand, consider investing in a food processor. A pressure cooker like the Instant Pot can significantly cut down on the time required to cook meats, bone broths, and one-pot meals. A slow cooker like a Crockpot allows you to safely leave meals cooking while you're away from the house. A spiralizer can be used to easily make Paleo pasta like zoodles (zucchini noodles).

5. **Go nuts.** Keep a variety of nuts on hand as a quick snack. This can help take the edge off when you're experiencing cravings, and also provide a healthy bite in a pinch. Limit consumption of nuts to no more than one handful per day. Eat a variety of nuts and seeds to avoid developing intolerance to any one type.

Your Paleo Kitchen

Now that you've purged your kitchen to make it Paleo, let's ensure that you have the essential supplies on hand. With these basic tools and staples, you'll find that cooking healthy Paleo foods is a lot easier than you thought.

Keep your pantry, refrigerator, and freezer stocked with these Paleo staples to save yourself time and money on your Paleo diet. Having these at arm's reach will minimize your time spent at the grocery store and in the kitchen.

PANTRY

Apple cider vinegar is a popular acid used in Paleo cooking. Drinking ½ cup water with 1 teaspoon apple cider vinegar stirred in 15 minutes before meals can also improve protein digestion.

Coconut aminos are a Paleo version of soy sauce made from the fermented sap of the coconut blossom. They can be found in health food stores and online.

Collagen powder (peptides) has no taste, dissolves in hot or cold liquid, and provides your daily dose of collagen, an important nutrient for skin, hair, nails, and more.

Full-fat coconut milk imparts a creaminess to dishes and is sold in BPA-free cans. Coconut cream is the fatty portion that rises to the top of a can of full-fat coconut milk (it can also be purchased on its own).

Garlic is another frequently used ingredient. You can purchase peeled garlic cloves and jarred or frozen minced garlic to save yourself time.

Onions are used in several recipes. Always have a few white or yellow onions and at least one red onion on hand.

Paleo cooking fats like coconut oil, extra-virgin olive oil, avocado oil, and grass-fed ghee are healthy alternatives to traditional oils. You can use these fats interchangeably in most recipes.

Salt and pepper are used in most recipes. We recommend using unrefined sea salt and freshly ground black pepper.

Eggs are protein powerhouses. Always have at least a dozen on hand for recipes, snacks, and baking.

Nuts are a handy snack in a pinch. Choose almonds, macadamia, cashews, walnuts, pecans, hazelnuts, pistachios, Brazil, and other raw or roasted nuts. Make sure no oils or other non-Paleo ingredients have been added. Store nuts in the refrigerator to keep them fresh and protect their delicate fats.

Nut butter, such as almond and cashew, makes a great snack when smeared on fruit or veggies. Store nut butters in the refrigerator once opened.

Nut or seed milks can be added to smoothies, coffee, tea, granola, and anywhere else you would use dairy milk. Almond, cashew, hemp, coconut, macadamia, and other dairy-free milks can be found in both the refrigerated and unrefrigerated sections of grocery stores.

Paleo mayonnaise is made from avocado or coconut oils. Once opened, it must be stored in the refrigerator. You can also make your own (see page 163).

Sparkling water without any additives makes for a thirst-quenching treat that can help break a dependency on soda, juice, or other sugar-laden beverages.

FREEZER

Bacon is like Paleo candy. Be sure you are purchasing a healthy, preservative-free variety and keep a few packs in your freezer for a quick breakfast or snack.

Chicken breasts or thighs are a meat staple that can be purchased in bulk and frozen to save money.

Frozen berries are convenient for making smoothies, dressings, sauces, and more.

Ground beef is a base for endless easy Paleo meals.

Salmon is loaded with anti-inflammatory omega-3 fatty acids. Stock up when it's in season and keep a fillet or two in your freezer.

Paleo baking flours like almond flour, coconut flour, tapioca flour/starch, and arrowroot flour/starch/powder can be used to make virtually any type of baked good that you desire. Buying these in bulk and storing them in the freezer is the most economical.

ESSENTIAL TOOLS AND EQUIPMENT

Whether you're a Paleo newbie or a seasoned pro, the right cookware can make or break your food preparation efforts. To minimize toxins leaching from cookware during cooking and cleaning, opt for stainless steel, glass, ceramic, silicone, or wood, and avoid plastic whenever possible.

Skillets (2). You'll want at least two of these, one large and one medium. Although nonstick varieties make cleanup easier, most nonstick coatings (like Teflon) can release potentially carcinogenic chemicals when they are overheated, scratched, or chipped. Stainless-steel or cast-iron skillets are preferable.

Saucepans/pots (2). You'll want a few different pots—at the very least, you'll need a large pot for making soups and bone broth and a small or medium pot for heating smaller volumes.

Baking sheet. A rimmed baking sheet or pan is useful for preparing one-pan dishes, baked goods, and more.

Baking dish. A large baking dish can be used to bake casseroles, frittatas, and cakes. Opt for ceramic or glass, if possible.

Muffin tin. A standard 12-cup muffin tin, lined with unbleached parchment paper baking cups, is handy for baking muffins, cupcakes, and egg bites. Silicone muffin cups are another nontoxic option.

Blender. Blenders are used to puree soups, sauces, smoothies, dressings, marinades, and more. Opt for a glass blender, which won't leach chemicals when you are blending hot substances.

Knives. Having a few different knives, such as a chef's knife and a paring knife, is essential for prepping all types of Paleo food.

Cutting board. You will use a large cutting board nearly every day to prep veggies, meats, and other ingredients.

Tongs. Tongs are very handy for flipping bacon and handling hot items.

Vegetable peeler. In addition to removing the skins from veggies, a handheld veggie peeler can be used to create strands of vegetables to imitate noodles.

Steamer basket. Although not essential, steamer baskets are inexpensive and make steaming vegetables a breeze.

Storage containers. Having containers of different sizes is essential for storing leftovers, taking Paleo foods on the go, and meal prepping. Opt for glass containers with airtight lids to minimize chemical leaching and keep your food fresher longer. Food-grade silicone bags are a healthy alternative to plastic zip-top bags.

Parchment paper. Unbleached parchment paper is used to line baking sheets when baking Paleo goods, and also makes for quick cleanup when you're making one-pan meals by preventing food from sticking to the pan.

PALEO-FRIENDLY SWAPS

NOT SO FRIENDLY	PALEO-FRIENDLY
Cooking oils (vegetable, canola, corn, soy, grapeseed, sunflower, safflower, etc.)	Extra-virgin olive oil, avocado oil, grass-fed ghee, and coconut oil
Dairy milk	Unsweetened coconut milk, almond milk, and other nut and seed milks
Wheat flour, all-purpose flour, and other grain-based flours	Almond flour and meal, coconut flour, tapioca flour, cassava flour, and other grain-free flours and starches
Dairy yogurt	Coconut, cashew, almond, and other dairy-free yogurts
Refined sugar	Raw honey, maple syrup, coconut sugar, dates, molasses, and other natural sweeteners
Peanut butter	Almond, cashew, and other nut and seed butters
Rice	Cauliflower Rice (page 70)
Soy sauce	Coconut aminos
Cornstarch	Arrowroot flour/starch/powder or tapioca flour/starch
Pasta	Zoodles (zucchini noodles; page 62) or baked spaghetti squash (see tip, page 129)
Salad dressings with non-Paleo oils	Extra-virgin olive oil and balsamic or apple cider vinegar
Grain-based breads	Grain-free bread (page 161)
Grain-based cereals and granolas	Grain-free cereal (page 57) and grain-free granola (page 156)

FAVORITE PALEO BRANDS

Purchasing premade ingredients can be a real time- and energy-saver. Here are some of our favorite companies and brands producing healthy Paleo-friendly staples. These products can be found in many major grocery stores, natural food stores, and online.

AIP (autoimmune protocol) prepared foods: Nowadays you can purchase pre-made AIP-friendly ingredients, snacks, and meals. Check out Thrive Market, Wild Zora, and Paleo On The Go.

Bone broth: Many store-bought bone broths are actually flavored water in disguise. Kettle & Fire makes shelf-stable, grass-fed, organic bone broths that are loaded with gut-healing collagen.

Paleo mayo: Paleo mayonnaise is made with avocado or coconut oil instead of vegetable oil. Although you can make your own (page 163), you can purchase Paleo mayo at many grocery stores and online. Our go-to brands are Chosen Foods, Primal Kitchen, and Sir Kensington's.

Condiments: Some of our favorite brands of healthier ketchup, mustard, and salad dressings are Sir Kensington's, Primal Kitchen, and Tessemae's.

Riced cauliflower: Stores like Trader Joe's and Costco now sell premade cauliflower rice, fresh and frozen.

Baked goods: Simple Mills makes delicious grain-free baking mixes for muffins, cakes, pancakes, pizza crusts, and breads.

Paleo tortillas, chips, and crackers: Siete Family Foods sells authentic grain-free tortillas and chips. Simple Mills has a variety of different grain-free crackers. Jackson's sweet potato chips are made with coconut and avocado oils, making them Paleo (in moderation!).

Grain-free granola: There are several brands of grain-free granola; just be sure to read the ingredients to ensure everything is Paleo-friendly. Check out Bubba's Fine Foods, Wildway, and Paleonola.

continued →

Paleo jerky: Always read ingredient labels, as many types of jerky are not Paleo. Epic, Paleovalley, and Chomps are reputable brands making Paleo jerky, meat bars, and other protein-packed snacks.

Protein bars: Epic, Lärabar, Bulletproof, and RXBar are companies that make Paleo-friendly protein bars for convenient snacks on the go.

Protein/collagen powder: Most protein powders are not Paleo, but ones with protein derived from meat, egg, seeds, or nuts are. Our favorite brand of collagen is Vital Proteins.

About the Recipes

Now that you're familiar with Paleo foods, how to shop, and how to avoid common Paleo pitfalls, let's shift gears and talk about the delicious recipes you'll be enjoying. Even if you don't fancy yourself a good cook, by the end of this journey, you'll be confident in the kitchen and well on your way to looking and feeling better than you have in years. The recipes in this book are designed with beginners (and flavor) in mind, and you'll notice some recurring themes:

Simple, budget-friendly meals. Simple ingredients, when combined correctly, make for delicious and satisfying meals. Fewer ingredients also make eating healthy a lot easier on your budget, and your digestion.

Easiness labels. Many of the recipes in this book fall into categories that indicate how easy they are to make and are labeled as follows:

 One main piece of cookware (one pot, one pan, one baking dish)

 Five ingredients or fewer

 30 minutes or less

 Superfast (10 minutes or less)

Smart tips. Most recipes feature tips that will save you additional time and money. They include:

- **Smart Shopping** tips suggest ways to save you money and help you identify the best Paleo brands to swap in.

- **Switch It Up** tips illustrate how easy it is to customize recipes with ingredients you prefer or have on hand.

- **Technique** tips give advice on things like how to make your own cauliflower rice and quick prep for other ingredients.

- **Love Your Leftovers** tips show you how to use up ingredients or leftovers.

Dietary labels identify recipes that follow AIP or that are egg-free, nut-free, vegan, vegetarian, or no-cook.

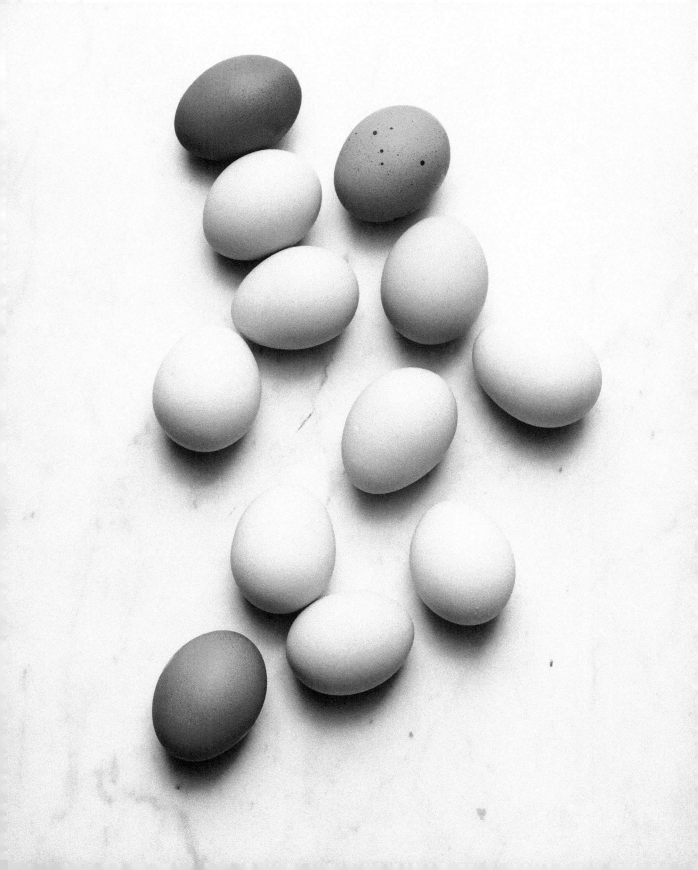

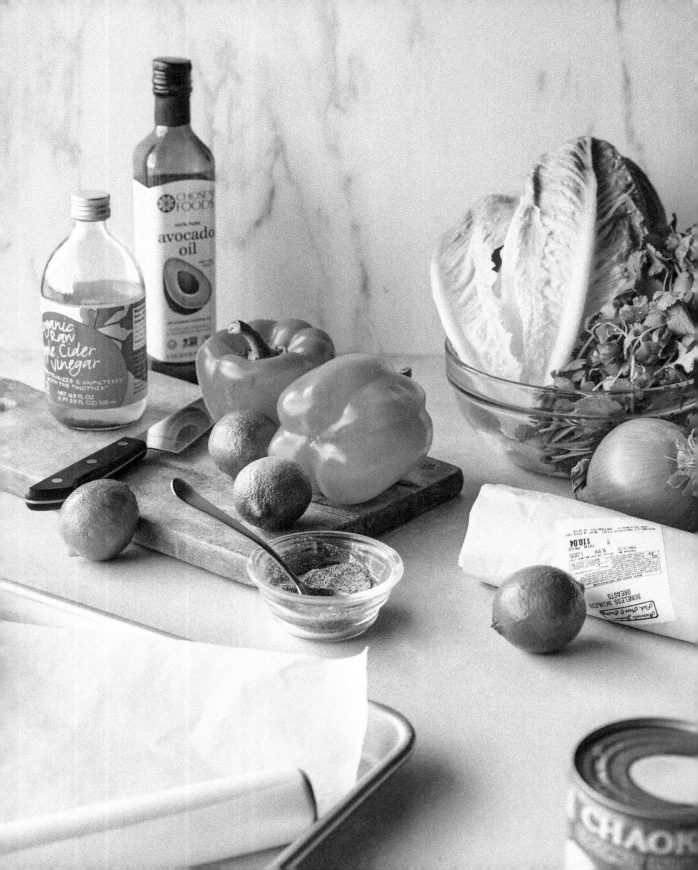

CHAPTER 2

Paleo Meal Plans

Now it's time to, quite literally, dig into the meat and potatoes of the diet. This chapter contains your road map to reaching your goals on the Paleo diet, whether that's losing weight, improving your overall health, or healing from a chronic condition. Here you'll find three Paleo meal plans that address different needs. The first was developed for readers who are new to meal planning, the second focuses on weight loss, and the third is for those interested in autoimmune protocol (AIP) benefits. Each 14-day plan includes shopping lists and prep tips. Later chapters in the book contain all the recipes for the meal plans, plus even more recipes to help you keep eating Paleo for the long run.

About the Plans

Your health journey is unique. That's why you'll find three different two-week meal plans in this chapter. If you're new to Paleo, we recommend the **Getting Started** plan. Consider the **Weight Loss** plan if you have a lot of weight to lose or want to include daily breakfast recipes in your meal plan. If you have an autoimmune disease or another inflammatory condition, you might want to jump right into the **Autoimmune Protocol (AIP)** meal plan. You really can't go wrong; all plans support weight loss, inflammation reduction, and an empowering move away from processed foods.

Getting Started: If you're not sure where to start, this is a great introduction to the other two plans in the book. Grab-and-go breakfasts and dinner leftovers make this the easiest plan to follow. The recipes are simple, and most take 30 minutes or less and use ingredients you may already have on hand.

Weight Loss: On this plan, you'll be cooking breakfast and dinner recipes for each day. To save time, you'll enjoy dinner leftovers for lunch most days. To expedite weight loss, you'll minimize high-glycemic fruit (e.g., bananas) and starchy vegetables (e.g., sweet potatoes, squash). Instead, opt for low-sugar fruits like berries and melons. You can easily swap nonstarchy veggies (e.g., zucchini, cauliflower, greens) into recipes.

Autoimmune Protocol (AIP): This plan also utilizes grab-and-go breakfasts and dinner leftovers for lunch. It is the most restrictive plan because additional items are excluded. Along with non-Paleo foods, you will also avoid nuts, seeds, eggs, nightshade vegetables, alcohol, ghee, sweeteners, and food additives. These foods include nut- and seed-derived items such as butters and flours, coffee, chocolate, seed oils (e.g., sesame oil), and seed-based spices (e.g., cumin). You will also remove nightshade-based spices, including cayenne, chili powder, paprika, curry powder, and others. Some people feel best if they also remove black pepper.

You will be adapting many recipes to make them AIP-friendly. Don't worry—it's easy! Check the weekly prep sections for instructions. You can simply omit non-AIP ingredients or sub in AIP-friendly alternatives. For instance, swap in zucchini for bell peppers, which are nightshades. The AIP is intended to be a temporary diet to facilitate gut healing and inflammation reduction. As you start feeling better, try slowly reintroducing the excluded foods one at a time.

Meal Plan Notes

The meal plans are designed so that you'll go grocery shopping on the weekends. If you already have items listed on the shopping lists, simply cross them off each week to avoid buying more than you need.

You will be meal prepping twice a week, we recommend Sundays and Wednesdays, but you can choose any days that work best for your schedule.

SERVING GUIDANCE

Each meal plan is designed for two average adults. If you're conquering Paleo on your own, simply cut the recipe and shopping list quantities in half. Recipes in the meal plan with a serving size of two will have no leftovers. Recipes that serve four will have leftovers that will be utilized at a later date. On Sundays, you will "graze the refrigerator for leftovers," which is an opportunity to use up any extra items so that nothing goes to waste. If you don't have any leftovers, use it as a chance to practice your Paleo dining-out skills!

FOOD STORAGE

If you have leftovers, most can be stored in airtight containers in the refrigerator for up to four days. We recommend glass containers with tight-fitting lids, which are convenient for reheating leftovers in the microwave. Plastic should never be heated in the microwave, as it can leach chemicals into your food.

MAKING SUBSTITUTIONS

Unless you have a known food intolerance or other reason you need to avoid a particular food, we encourage you to follow the meal plans as written, as they have been specifically designed to maximize your results while eating Paleo. Optimal health requires the inclusion of a wide variety of foods in your diet. Likewise, food intolerance can develop when we consume the same foods over and over again. Be willing to try new foods and revisit ones you had written out of your life.

Having said that, nearly every ingredient in the recipes can be easily swapped out by substituting a similar food of the same quantity. For example, if you don't eat pork, replace it with another type of meat of the same amount listed in the recipe and shopping list. Or perhaps you don't like tomatoes or bell peppers. Simply choose a different vegetable to use in recipes that call for them. You may need to adjust cook times. If you avoid eggs, it will be easiest to swap out recipes that are egg-based and replace them with different, egg-free dishes.

A NOTE ON SNACKS

Although snacks aren't included in the meal plan, you are welcome to snack between meals. Some people find Paleo meals more filling and don't feel the need to snack, whereas others are hungrier during the transition. Let your appetite guide you, but be sure you're snacking for the right reasons, not because you're bored, tired, or emotional. Keep in mind that thirst is often disguised as hunger. Stay hydrated by drinking enough water each day. For most people, drinking half your weight (in pounds) in ounces of water will be sufficient: if you weigh 200 pounds, for example, aim to drink about 100 ounces of water per day.

The following grab-and-go snack options make snacking easy, fast, and healthy. You're also welcome to make your own snacks using the recipes in the snacks chapter (chapter 8). You'll be more satisfied if you opt for proteins and fats over carbohydrates. Always pair carb snacks with protein and/or fat—smear some almond butter on that apple!

GRAB-AND-GO SNACKS

*Autoimmune protocol (AIP)–friendly snacks are noted with an asterisk. When purchasing prepared items, ensure that all ingredients are AIP-compliant.

1. Small handful of nuts (about ¼ cup)

2. 1 to 2 ounces beef jerky (see brands on page 17), 2 cooked bacon slices*, or a single serving of deli meat*

3. ½ apple* and 2 tablespoons almond butter

4. ½ cup berries or orange slices with 1 tablespoon coconut cream or 2 tablespoons coconut butter*

5. 5 to 10 olives*

6. ½ avocado with sea salt and lime or topped with ½ can sardines, salmon, or tuna*

7. 2 dates with 1 tablespoon coconut butter*

8. 1 hard-boiled egg with sea salt and freshly ground black pepper

9. ½ baked sweet potato stuffed with 1 tablespoon coconut oil or coconut cream and/or ½ can tuna or salmon*

10. 2 ounces smoked salmon or lox with 1 ounce plantain chips*

Meal Plan 1: Getting Started

Welcome to your first week of Paleo! The Getting Started plan introduces you to Paleo while saving you time in the kitchen. The weekly prep gets you through a five-day workweek. You can prep ahead for weekends or cook food fresh on Saturdays. You'll save time with simple breakfasts and dinner leftovers for lunch. Make entire meals in advance or prep meals in part (e.g., assemble sauces, chop veggies) to make mealtime a breeze.

	Breakfast	Lunch	Dinner
MONDAY	Per person: 4 bacon slices + 2 eggs + 1 serving fruit of choice	Easy Tuna Salad	One-Pan Chicken and Chard
TUESDAY	Per person: 4 bacon slices + 2 eggs + 1 serving fruit of choice	Leftover One-Pan Chicken and Chard	Beef-tastic Tacos + Simple Cauliflower Rice
WEDNESDAY	Good Day Green Smoothie	Leftover Beef-tastic Tacos + Simple Cauliflower Rice	Southwest Chorizo Stew
THURSDAY	Per person: ½ avocado + 2 ounces lox + ¼ cup nuts	Leftover Southwest Chorizo Stew	Steak with Mango Salsa
FRIDAY	Per person: ½ avocado + 2 ounces lox + ¼ cup nuts	Leftover Steak with Mango Salsa	Red Curry Cod
SATURDAY	Almond Banana Pancakes with Blackberry Sauce	Leftover Red Curry Cod	Chicken Veggie Stir-Fry
SUNDAY	Leftover Almond Banana Pancakes with Blackberry Sauce	Graze the refrigerator for leftovers	Leftover Chicken Veggie Stir-Fry

WEEK 1 SHOPPING LIST

PANTRY

- Apple cider vinegar
- Baking soda
- Black pepper, ground
- Cayenne pepper
- Chili powder
- Chipotle chile, ground
- Cumin, ground
- Dill, dried
- Flour, almond
- Flour, tapioca
- Garlic powder
- Oil, avocado
- Oil, toasted sesame
- Onion powder
- Sea salt
- Vanilla extract, pure

SHELF-STABLE

- Chicken broth (5½ cups)
- Coconut aminos (2 tablespoons)
- Collagen powder (¼ cup)
- Curry paste, red (5 tablespoons)
- Milk, almond (1 cup)
- Milk, coconut, full-fat (one 13.5-ounce can)
- Nuts, any type (1 cup)
- Paleo mayonnaise (⅓ cup)

PRODUCE

- Avocados (3½)
- Bananas (3)
- Bell peppers, any color (2)
- Blueberries (1 cup)
- Bok choy, baby (1 pound)
- Broccoli (4 cups florets)
- Carrot (1)
- Cauliflower (1 head, or 4 cups riced)
- Celery (2 stalks)
- Chard (1 bunch)
- Cilantro (2 bunches)
- Fruit of choice (4 servings)
- Garlic (6 cloves)
- Ginger, fresh (one ½-inch piece)
- Grapes, green (2 cups)
- Green beans (¼ pound)
- Greens, mixed (4 cups)
- Kale, any type (2 bunches)
- Lemon (1)
- Limes (1½)
- Lettuce, romaine (8 leaves)
- Mangos (2)
- Mushrooms (1 cup sliced)
- Onion, red (1)
- Onion, yellow or white (1)
- Parsley (1 bunch)
- Scallions (2)
- Sweet potatoes (3)
- Tomatoes (3)

MEAT, FISH, AND EGGS

- Bacon (16 slices)
- Beef, flank steak (1½ pounds)
- Beef, ground (1½ pounds)
- Chicken, cooked, homemade or rotisserie (3 cups)
- Chicken, thighs, bone-in, skin-on (4)
- Chorizo (1 pound)
- Cod (1½ pounds)
- Eggs, large (12)
- Lox (8 ounces)
- Tuna, oil- or water-packed (two 5-ounce cans)

WEEK 1 PREP

ON SUNDAY

1. For Monday and Tuesday breakfasts, cook the bacon (16 slices) and hard-boil 8 eggs. If desired, wash and prep your fruit of choice.

2. For Monday lunch, make the *Easy Tuna Salad* (page 82).

3. For Monday dinner, prep the veggies for *One-Pan Chicken and Chard* (page 112).

4. For Tuesday dinner, cook the meat with the spice blend for *Beef-tastic Tacos* (page 127). Rice the cauliflower for *Simple Cauliflower Rice* (page 70; skip this if you purchased riced cauliflower instead).

5. For Wednesday breakfast, prep the ingredients for *Good Day Green Smoothie* (page 52) and place them in a freezer container, minus the liquid. Freeze so it's ready to heat and eat.

6. For Wednesday dinner, prep the veggies for *Southwest Chorizo Stew* (page 143).

ON WEDNESDAY

1. If desired, for Thursday and Friday breakfasts, portion out the lox and nuts.

2. For Thursday dinner, make the salsa for *Steak with Mango Salsa* (page 136).

3. For Friday dinner, prep the kale for *Red Curry Cod* (page 86).

4. Optional: For Saturday breakfast, prep the sauce for *Almond Banana Pancakes with Blackberry Sauce* (page 50). You can also prepare the pancakes in advance, so they're ready to heat and eat.

5. Optional: For Saturday dinner, prepare the *Chicken Veggie Stir-Fry* (page 114), or just prep the veggies for the stir-fry.

Congratulations on conquering your first week of Paleo! Truth be told, you might not be feeling 100 percent this week. Headaches, bowel changes, fatigue, and irritability are all common. These are reassuring signs that you really needed this change. Be patient with your body as it detoxes years of stored toxins and transitions into a fat-burning machine. Get plenty of rest, daily movement, and ample hydration to speed the detox process along. Make your kitchen prep time more fun by listening to music or your favorite podcast!

	Breakfast	Lunch	Dinner
MONDAY	Grab-and-Go Egg Bites	Ham and Baby Kale Salad	So-Good Sloppy Joes
TUESDAY	Leftover Grab-and-Go Egg Bites	Leftover So-Good Sloppy Joes	Turkey Burgers on Portobello Buns
WEDNESDAY	Very Berry Smoothie	Leftover Turkey Burgers on Portobello Buns	Shrimp Scampi with Zoodles
THURSDAY	Per person: ½ avocado + 2 ounces turkey slices + ¼ cup nuts	Leftover Shrimp Scampi with Zoodles	Pork Fried Rice
FRIDAY	Per person: ½ avocado + 2 ounces turkey slices + ¼ cup nuts	Leftover Pork Fried Rice	Butternut Bacon-Wrapped Chicken Thighs
SATURDAY	Sausage Frittata	Leftover Butternut Bacon-Wrapped Chicken Thighs	"Spaghetti" and Meatballs
SUNDAY	Leftover Sausage Frittata	Graze the refrigerator for leftovers	Leftover "Spaghetti" and Meatballs

PANTRY

- Apple cider vinegar
- Black pepper, ground
- Chili powder
- Chipotle chile, ground
- Cinnamon, ground
- Cumin, ground
- Garlic powder
- Ghee, grass-fed
- Italian seasoning
- Mustard, Dijon
- Oil, avocado
- Oil, extra-virgin olive
- Oil, toasted sesame
- Onion powder
- Red pepper flakes
- Sea salt

SHELF-STABLE

- Chicken broth (⅓ cup)
- Coconut aminos (3 tablespoons)
- Collagen powder (¼ cup)
- Marinara sauce (one 25-ounce jar)
- Milk, almond (1½ cups)
- Milk, coconut, full-fat, canned (⅓ cup)
- Nuts, any type (1 cup)
- Paleo mayonnaise (½ cup)
- Tomato sauce (one 15-ounce can)

PRODUCE

- Arugula (2 cups)
- Avocados (3)
- Banana (1)
- Bell pepper, any color (1)
- Berries, any type, frozen (2 cups)
- Broccoli (1 cup florets)
- Butternut squash (1)
- Carrots (2)
- Cauliflower (1 head or 4 cups riced)
- Celery (2 stalks)
- Chard (1 bunch)
- Garlic (6 cloves)
- Ginger, fresh (1 tablespoon grated)
- Kale, any type (1 bunch)
- Kale, baby (6 cups)
- Lemon (½)
- Lime (1)
- Mushrooms, portobello caps (4)
- Onions, yellow or white (3)
- Parsley (1 bunch)
- Spaghetti squash (1)
- Sweet potato (1)
- Tomatoes (4)
- Zucchini (4)

MEAT, FISH, AND EGGS

- Bacon (8 slices)
- Bacon, Canadian (7 ounces)
- Beef, ground (2 pounds)
- Chicken, thighs, bone-in or boneless, skinless (8)
- Eggs, large (20)
- Ham, cooked (8 ounces)
- Pork, ground (1 pound)
- Sausage, ground (½ pound)
- Shrimp, large, peeled and deveined (1½ pounds)
- Turkey, deli slices, (8 ounces)
- Turkey, ground (1½ pounds)

ON SUNDAY

1. For Monday breakfast, prepare *Grab-and-Go Egg Bites* (page 54).

2. For Monday lunch, prepare *Ham and Baby Kale Salad* (page 126). Store the salad and dressing separately until ready to serve.

3. For Monday dinner, prepare *So-Good Sloppy Joes* (page 128), or just prep the veggies for the sloppy joes.

4. For Tuesday dinner, prep the veggies, assemble the turkey patties, and make the mayo for *Turkey Burgers on Portobello Buns* (page 111).

5. For Wednesday breakfast, prep the ingredients for *Very Berry Smoothie* (page 58) and place them in a freezer container, minus the liquid. Freeze so it's ready for you to add liquid and blend.

6. For Wednesday dinner, prep the shrimp, zoodles, and veggies for *Shrimp Scampi with Zoodles* (page 88).

ON WEDNESDAY

1. If desired, for Thursday and Friday breakfasts, portion out the turkey and nuts.

2. For Thursday dinner, prep the veggies for *Pork Fried Rice* (page 134).

3. For Friday dinner, peel and chop the butternut squash for *Butternut Bacon-Wrapped Chicken Thighs* (page 109).

4. Optional: For Saturday breakfast, prepare the *Sausage Frittata* (page 56).

5. Optional: For Saturday dinner, cook the squash and assemble the *"Spaghetti" and Meatballs* (page 129), or just cook the meatballs.

Meal Plan 2: Weight Loss

Welcome to the Weight Loss meal plan. Get ready to enjoy mouthwatering meals as you eat your way to vibrant health! This adventure is more than just a diet—it's a lifestyle. Paleo includes daily movement, hydration, restorative sleep, and community. Try giving each of these attention this week. *Bon appétit!*

	Breakfast	Lunch	Dinner
MONDAY	Grab-and-Go Egg Bites	Smoked Salmon Lettuce Rolls	Kickin' Chicken Strips + Cauliflower Mash
TUESDAY	Berry Protein Muffins	Leftover Kickin' Chicken Strips + Cauliflower Mash	So-Good Sloppy Joes
WEDNESDAY	Leftover Grab-and-Go Egg Bites	Leftover So-Good Sloppy Joes	Sheet Pan Fajitas with Coconut-Lime Dressing
THURSDAY	Leftover Berry Protein Muffins	Leftover Sheet Pan Fajitas with Coconut-Lime Dressing	"Spaghetti" and Meatballs
FRIDAY	Very Berry Smoothie	Leftover "Spaghetti" and Meatballs	Fiesta Fish Tacos
SATURDAY	Nutty Paleo Cereal	Leftover Fiesta Fish Tacos	Pulled Pork
SUNDAY	Leftover Nutty Paleo Cereal	Graze the refrigerator for leftovers	Leftover Pulled Pork

PANTRY

- Apple cider vinegar
- Black pepper, ground
- Baking soda
- Chili powder
- Cinnamon, ground
- Cumin, ground
- Flour, almond
- Flour, tapioca
- Garlic powder
- Ghee
- Honey
- Italian seasoning
- Mustard, Dijon
- Oil, avocado
- Oil, coconut
- Onion powder
- Paprika
- Sea salt
- Taco seasoning
- Vanilla extract, pure

SHELF-STABLE

- Almonds, chopped (1 cup)
- Apples, dried, unsweetened (½ cup)
- Chicken broth (1 cup)
- Coconut aminos (1 teaspoon)
- Coconut flakes, unsweetened (1 cup)
- Collagen powder (¾ cup)
- Marinara sauce (one 25-ounce jar)
- Milk, almond (1¾ cups)
- Milk, coconut, full-fat, canned (½ cup)
- Sriracha (1½ teaspoons)
- Sunflower seeds, hulled (½ cup)
- Tahini (¼ cup)
- Tomato sauce (one 15-ounce can)

PRODUCE

- Avocados (2)
- Banana (1)
- Bell peppers, any color (3½)
- Berries, any type, frozen (2 cups)
- Blueberries (2½ cups)
- Broccoli (1 cup florets)
- Cabbage, any color (⅛ head)
- Carrots (4)
- Cauliflower (1 head or 4 cups riced)
- Celery (6 stalks)
- Chard (1 bunch)
- Cilantro (2 bunches)
- Garlic (4 cloves)
- Lemon (1)
- Lettuce, butter (8 leaves)
- Lettuce, romaine (2 heads)
- Limes (3)
- Onion, red (½)
- Onions, yellow or white (3)
- Parsnips (4)
- Spaghetti squash (1)

MEAT, FISH, AND EGGS

- Bacon, Canadian (7 ounces)
- Beef, ground (2 pounds)
- Chicken breast, boneless, skinless (1½ pounds)
- Cod (1 pound)
- Eggs, large (14)
- Pork, shoulder roast (4 pounds)
- Salmon, smoked (6 ounces)
- Turkey breast, boneless, skinless (1 pound)

WEEK 1 PREP

ON SUNDAY

1. For Monday breakfast, make *Grab-and-Go Egg Bites* (page 54).

2. For Monday lunch, make *Smoked Salmon Lettuce Rolls* (page 95).

3. For Monday dinner, prepare *Cauliflower Mash* (page 72). If desired, prepare *Kickin' Chicken Strips* (page 108) so they're ready to heat and eat.

4. For Tuesday breakfast, make *Berry Protein Muffins* (page 53).

5. For Tuesday dinner, make *So-Good Sloppy Joes* (page 128) or prep just the veggies.

6. For Wednesday dinner, prepare the dressing, make the spice blend, and prep the veggies and turkey for *Sheet Pan Fajitas with Coconut-Lime Dressing* (page 115).

ON WEDNESDAY

1. For Thursday dinner, cook the squash and assemble or cook the meatballs for *"Spaghetti" and Meatballs* (page 129).

2. For Friday breakfast, prep the ingredients for *Very Berry Smoothie* (page 58) and place them in a freezer container, minus the liquid. Freeze so they're ready for you to add liquid and blend.

3. For Friday dinner, prepare the slaw for *Fiesta Fish Tacos* (page 98).

4. Optional: For Saturday breakfast, make *Nutty Paleo Cereal* (page 57).

5. Optional: For Saturday dinner, assemble the ingredients for *Pulled Pork* (page 141) in the slow cooker insert and refrigerate. Start slow cooking Saturday morning.

On the cellular level, it takes a few weeks for your body to learn how to burn fat for fuel. This is known as becoming "fat-adapted" or "keto-adapted." Once your body shifts from burning sugar (glucose) to primarily using fat (ketones) for energy, weight loss becomes much easier. If you experience sugar cravings, drink a glass of water, take a walk, or enjoy a fat- or protein-based snack instead.

	Breakfast	Lunch	Dinner
MONDAY	Spinach and Shroom Scramble	Turkey Wraps	Butternut Bacon-Wrapped Chicken Thighs
TUESDAY	Almond Banana Pancakes with Blackberry Sauce	Leftover Butternut Bacon-Wrapped Chicken Thighs	Pepper Steak with Cilantro Rice
WEDNESDAY	Leftover Spinach and Shroom Scramble	Leftover Pepper Steak with Cilantro Rice	Breaded Pork Chops with Green Apple Slaw
THURSDAY	Leftover Almond Banana Pancakes with Blackberry Sauce	Leftover Breaded Pork Chops with Green Apple Slaw	Turkey Burgers on Portobello Buns
FRIDAY	Good Day Green Smoothie	Leftover Turkey Burgers on Portobello Buns	Baked Salmon Cakes + Garlicky Creamed Greens
SATURDAY	Chorizo Hash	Leftover Baked Salmon Cakes + Garlicky Creamed Greens	Perfect Paleo Chili
SUNDAY	Leftover Chorizo Hash	Graze the refrigerator for leftovers	Leftover Perfect Paleo Chili

PANTRY

- Apple cider vinegar
- Black pepper, ground
- Baking soda
- Chili powder
- Chipotle chile, ground
- Cumin, ground
- Flour, almond
- Flour, coconut
- Flour, tapioca
- Garlic powder
- Ghee
- Italian seasoning
- Mustard, Dijon
- Oil, avocado
- Oil, coconut
- Onion powder
- Red pepper flakes
- Sea salt
- Vanilla extract, pure

SHELF-STABLE

- Coconut aminos (¼ cup)
- Collagen powder (¼ cup)
- Dill pickle slices (⅓ cup)
- Milk, almond (1 cup)
- Milk, coconut, full-fat, canned (⅔ cup)
- Paleo mayonnaise (¾ cup plus 2 tablespoons)
- Salmon (two 14-ounce cans)
- Tomatoes, fire-roasted, crushed (one 28-ounce can)

PRODUCE

- Apple, green (1)
- Arugula (2 cups)
- Avocado (½)
- Bananas (3)
- Basil (¼ cup)
- Bell peppers, any color (5)
- Blueberries (1 cup)
- Butternut squash (1)
- Cabbage, green (½ head)
- Cauliflower (2 heads, or 8 cups riced)
- Cilantro (1 bunch)
- Garlic (16 cloves)
- Ginger, fresh (1 tablespoon grated)
- Grapes, green (2 cups)
- Kale (1 bunch)
- Lemon (½)
- Lettuce (4 leaves)
- Limes (3)
- Mushrooms, button (4 cups sliced)
- Mushrooms, portobello (4 caps)
- Onion, red (1)
- Onions, yellow or white (2½)
- Parsley (1 bunch)
- Scallions (6)
- Spinach, baby (20 cups)
- Tomatoes (2)
- Tomatoes, Roma (4)

MEAT, FISH, AND EGGS

- Bacon (8 slices)
- Beef, ground (1 pound)
- Beef, steak, sirloin (1 pound)
- Chicken, thighs, bone-in or boneless, skinless (8)
- Chorizo, ground (12 ounces)
- Eggs, large (14)
- Pork chops, bone-in or boneless (4)
- Turkey, deli slices (8 ounces)
- Turkey, ground (1½ pounds)

ON SUNDAY

1. For Monday breakfast, prep *Spinach and Shroom Scramble* (page 47).

2. For Monday lunch, prep *Turkey Wraps* (page 110).

3. For Monday dinner, peel and chop the squash for *Butternut Bacon-Wrapped Chicken Thighs* (page 109).

4. For Tuesday breakfast, prep the sauce for *Almond Banana Pancakes with Blackberry Sauce* (page 50). You can also prepare the pancakes in advance, so they're ready to heat and eat.

5. For Tuesday dinner, prep the veggies for the steak and make the "rice" for *Pepper Steak with Cilantro Rice* (page 130).

6. For Wednesday dinner, shred the cabbage or make the slaw in full for *Breaded Pork Chops with Green Apple Slaw* (page 137).

ON WEDNESDAY

1. For Thursday dinner, prep the veggies, assemble the turkey patties, and make the mayo for *Turkey Burgers on Portobello Buns* (page 111).

2. For Friday breakfast, prep the ingredients for *Good Day Green Smoothie* (page 52) and place them in a freezer container, minus the liquid. Freeze so they're ready to add liquid and blend.

3. For Friday dinner, assemble the *Baked Salmon Cakes* (page 87) and refrigerate them until you are ready to bake.

4. Optional: For Saturday breakfast, make *Chorizo Hash* (page 46) or prep just the veggies.

5. Optional: For Saturday dinner, make *Perfect Paleo Chili* (page 132) or prep just the veggies.

Meal Plan 3: Autoimmune Protocol (AIP)

AIP is designed to jump-start gut healing and reduce inflammation. **Follow the weekly prep to make your recipes AIP-friendly.** Use Homemade Bone Broth (page 168) in recipes that call for broth.

	Breakfast	Lunch	Dinner
MONDAY	Per person: 4 bacon slices + ½ avocado + 1 orange	Ham and Baby Kale Salad	Halibut with Basil Coconut Cream + Garlicky Creamed Greens
TUESDAY	Per person: 4 bacon slices + ½ avocado + 1 orange	Leftover Halibut with Basil Coconut Cream + Garlicky Creamed Greens	Whole Roasted Chicken + Root Vegetable Puree
WEDNESDAY	Very Berry Smoothie	Leftover Whole Roasted Chicken + Root Vegetable Puree	"Spaghetti" and Meatballs
THURSDAY	Per person: ½ avocado + 2 ounces turkey slices + 1 apple	Leftover "Spaghetti" and Meatballs	Pork Fried Rice
FRIDAY	Per person: ½ avocado + 2 ounces turkey slices + 1 apple	Leftover Pork Fried Rice	Rosemary Lamb Chops with Olive Tapenade + Roasted Brussels Sprouts
SATURDAY	Meaty Breakfast Skillet	Leftover Rosemary Lamb Chops with Olive Tapenade + Roasted Brussels Sprouts	Butternut Bacon-Wrapped Chicken Thighs
SUNDAY	Leftover Meaty Breakfast Skillet	Graze the refrigerator for leftovers	Leftover Butternut Bacon-Wrapped Chicken Thighs

PANTRY

- Apple cider vinegar
- Black pepper, ground
- Cinnamon, ground
- Garlic powder
- Italian seasoning
- Oil, avocado
- Oil, coconut
- Oil, extra-virgin olive
- Onion powder
- Rosemary, dried
- Sea salt

SHELF-STABLE

- Chicken broth (½ cup)
- Coconut aminos (3 tablespoons)
- Collagen powder (¼ cup)
- Milk, coconut, full-fat, canned (1⅔ cups)
- Olives, green, pitted (1 cup)
- Olives, Kalamata, pitted (1 cup)

MEAT, FISH, AND EGGS

- Bacon (24 slices)
- Beef, ground (2 pounds)
- Chicken, thighs, bone-in or boneless, skinless (8)
- Chicken, whole (one 3½- to 5-pound bird)
- Halibut fillets (four 4- to 6-ounce pieces)
- Ham, cooked (8 ounces)
- Lamb, chops (2 pounds)
- Pork, ground (1 pound)
- Turkey, deli slices (8 ounces)

PRODUCE

- Apples (4)
- Avocados (5)
- Banana (1)
- Basil (1 bunch)
- Berries, fresh, any type (2 cups)
- Berries, frozen, any type (2 cups)
- Brussels sprouts (4 cups)
- Butternut squash (1)
- Carrots (7)
- Cauliflower (1 head or 4 cups riced)
- Garlic (14 cloves)
- Ginger, fresh (1 tablespoon grated)
- Jicama (1)
- Kale, baby (6 cups)
- Lemons (3½)
- Onion, yellow or white (1)
- Oranges (4)
- Parsley (1 bunch)
- Parsnips (4)
- Scallions (2)
- Spaghetti squash (1)
- Spinach, baby (20 cups)
- Tomatoes (2)
- Zucchini (1)

ON SUNDAY

1. For Monday and Tuesday breakfasts, cook the bacon (16 slices).

2. For Monday lunch, make *Ham and Baby Kale Salad* (page 126). **Replace the tomatoes with chopped jicama.** Keep the dressing separate until you are ready to serve.

3. For Monday dinner, prep the veggies for *Halibut with Basil Coconut Cream* (page 92) and *Garlicky Creamed Greens* (page 67). **Follow the tip in the halibut recipe to make AIP-friendly lemon pepper seasoning.**

4. For Tuesday dinner, prepare *Whole Roasted Chicken* (page 165) and *Root Vegetable Puree* (page 73).

5. For Wednesday breakfast, prep ingredients for *Very Berry Smoothie* (page 58) and place in a freezer container, minus the liquid. Freeze so it's ready to add liquid and blend. **When preparing the smoothie, omit the almond milk; use ½ cup full-fat coconut milk plus 1 cup water instead.**

6. For Wednesday dinner, cook the spaghetti squash and assemble or cook the meatballs for *"Spaghetti" and Meatballs* (page 129). **Omit the marinara sauce and drizzle with olive oil or purchase an AIP-friendly pasta sauce.**

ON WEDNESDAY

1. For Thursday dinner, prep the veggies for *Pork Fried Rice* (page 134). **Omit the eggs and sesame oil.**

2. For Friday dinner, make the olive tapenade for *Rosemary Lamb Chops with Olive Tapenade and Green Beans* (page 140). **Omit the green beans and serve with Brussels sprouts instead.** Prep the raw sprouts or make *Roasted Brussels Sprouts* (page 66).

3. Optional: For Saturday breakfast, use **ground beef** to prepare *Meaty Breakfast Skillet* (page 48).

4. Optional: For Saturday dinner, peel and chop the butternut squash for *Butternut Bacon-Wrapped Chicken Thighs* (page 109).

An unhealthy gut is at the root of most chronic inflammatory conditions, including autoimmunity. Consume seafood at least three times a week for anti-inflammatory omega-3 fatty acids. Use Homemade Bone Broth (page 168) in recipes that call for broth and sip some each morning for its gut-healing benefits.

	Breakfast	Lunch	Dinner
MONDAY	Per person: ½ avocado + 2 ounces lox + ½ cup berries	Puree of Pumpkin Soup + "Cheesy" Kale Chips	Shrimp Scampi with Zoodles
TUESDAY	Per person: ½ avocado + 2 ounces lox + ½ cup berries	Leftover Shrimp Scampi with Zoodles	Pepper Steak with Cilantro Rice
WEDNESDAY	Good Day Green Smoothie	Leftover Pepper Steak with Cilantro Rice	One-Pan Chicken and Chard
THURSDAY	Per person: 1 baked sweet potato + 3 tablespoons coconut cream + 4 bacon slices	Leftover One-Pan Chicken and Chard	Breaded Pork Chops with Green Apple Slaw
FRIDAY	Per person: 1 baked sweet potato + 3 tablespoons coconut cream + 4 bacon slices	Leftover Breaded Pork Chops with Green Apple Slaw	Coconut-Poached Sea Bass + Sweet Potato Fries
SATURDAY	Meaty Breakfast Skillet	Leftover Coconut-Poached Sea Bass + Sweet Potato Fries	Pulled Pork
SUNDAY	Leftover Meaty Breakfast Skillet	Graze the refrigerator for leftovers	Leftover Pulled Pork

PANTRY

- Apple cider vinegar
- Black pepper, ground
- Cinnamon, ground
- Garlic powder
- Ginger, ground
- Italian seasoning
- Oil, avocado
- Oil, coconut
- Oil, extra-virgin olive
- Onion powder
- Sea salt

SHELF-STABLE

- Chicken broth (3⅓ cups)
- Coconut aminos (¼ cup)
- Coconut cream (¾ cup)
- Coconut water (1 cup)
- Collagen powder (¼ cup)
- Milk, coconut, full-fat, canned (1 cup)
- Nutritional yeast (¼ cup)
- Pumpkin puree, pure (two 15-ounce cans)

MEAT, FISH, AND EGGS

- Bacon (16 slices)
- Beef, sirloin steak (1 pound)
- Chicken, thighs, bone-in, skin-on (4)
- Lox (8 ounces)
- Pork, chops, bone-in or boneless (4)
- Pork, shoulder roast, (4 pounds)
- Sea bass (four 4- to 6-ounce fillets)
- Shrimp, large, peeled and deveined (1½ pounds)
- Turkey, ground (1 pound)

PRODUCE

- Apple, green (1)
- Avocados (2½)
- Berries, any type, fresh (4 cups)
- Cabbage, green (½ head)
- Carrots (4)
- Cauliflower (1 head or 4 cups riced)
- Celery (4 stalks)
- Chard (1 bunch)
- Cilantro (1 bunch)
- Garlic (13 cloves)
- Ginger, fresh (1 tablespoon grated)
- Grapes, green (2 cups)
- Green (2)
- Kale, any type (1 bunch)
- Kale, curly (2 bunches)
- Lemon (½)
- Limes (2)
- Onions, yellow or white (3)
- Parsley (1 bunch)
- Parsnips (4)
- Scallions (2)
- Spinach, baby (4 cups)
- Sweet potatoes (8)
- Zucchini (7)

ON SUNDAY

1. For Monday lunch, prepare *Puree of Pumpkin Soup* (page 78). **Omit the optional pumpkin seeds.** Prepare *"Cheesy" Kale Chips* (page 151). **Freeze leftover soup or enjoy it with leftover kale chips for snacks.**

2. For Monday dinner, prep the zoodles, veggies, and shrimp for *Shrimp Scampi with Zoodles* (page 88). **Replace the ghee with olive oil. Omit the optional red pepper flakes.**

3. For Tuesday dinner, prep the steak veggies and make cilantro rice for *Pepper Steak with Cilantro Rice* (page 130). **Replace the bell peppers with 2 zucchini, sliced.**

4. For Wednesday breakfast, prep the ingredients for *Good Day Green Smoothie* (page 52), place in a freezer container, minus the liquid, and freeze. **When preparing the smoothie, replace the almond milk with coconut water.**

5. For Wednesday dinner, prep the veggies for *One-Pan Chicken and Chard* (page 112).

ON WEDNESDAY

1. For Thursday and Friday breakfasts, bake 4 sweet potatoes. Pierce each with a fork to allow steam to escape. Place on a foil-lined baking sheet. Bake at 425°F for 45 to 60 minutes, until tender when pierced. Cook the bacon (16 slices).

2. For Thursday dinner, shred the cabbage or make the slaw in full for *Breaded Pork Chops with Green Apple Slaw* (page 137). **Omit the almond flour from the pork.**

3. For Friday dinner, prep the raw sweet potatoes or entirely prepare *Sweet Potato Fries* (page 64).

4. Optional: For Saturday breakfast, use **ground turkey** to prepare *Meaty Breakfast Skillet* (page 48).

5. Optional: For Saturday dinner, assemble the ingredients for *Pulled Pork* (page 141) in the slow cooker insert, **omitting the paprika, chili powder, and cumin,** and refrigerate. Start slow cooking Saturday morning for dinner.

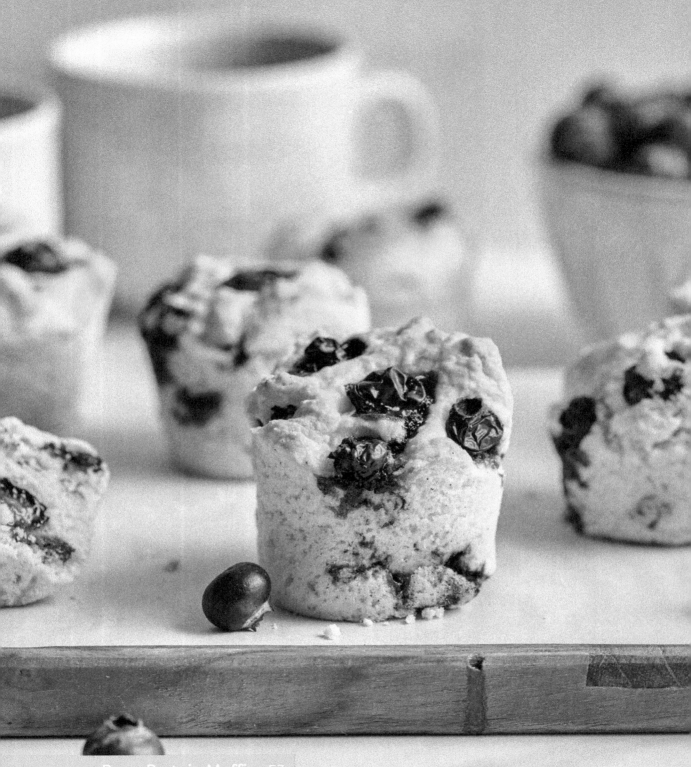

CHAPTER 3

Breakfast and Smoothies

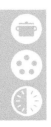

Chorizo Hash

Egg-Free, Nut-Free
Serves 4 / Prep time: 10 minutes **/ Cook time:** 10 minutes

For an extra protein punch, top this hash with a fried egg, or turn up the heat by adding chili powder, cayenne, or paprika. For variety, replace the cauliflower rice with sautéed diced sweet potatoes or white potatoes, which are Paleo-friendly when consumed in moderation.

12 ounces ground
   chorizo
1 bell pepper
½ medium onion
2 garlic cloves
1 large head
   cauliflower, or 4 cups
   riced cauliflower
¼ teaspoon sea salt
¼ teaspoon freshly
   ground black pepper

1. In a large pan, cook the chorizo over medium heat, stirring, until almost browned, about 4 minutes.

2. While the chorizo cooks, chop the bell pepper and onion into small, diced pieces. Mince the garlic. If using a head of cauliflower, break it into florets and put in a food processor. Pulse several times, until the cauliflower resembles grains of rice. (Alternatively, finely dice the cauliflower by hand or grate on the large holes of a box grater.)

3. Add the bell pepper, onion, garlic, salt, and pepper to the pan with the chorizo, and sauté for 1 to 2 more minutes. Add the riced cauliflower. Cook, stirring frequently, for 5 minutes. Enjoy!

Ingredient Tip: For this recipe, any type of ground meat, such as breakfast sausage, chicken, turkey, or beef, can be used in place of the chorizo.

Technique Tip: If you're starting with a whole head of cauliflower instead of riced cauliflower, break it into florets, then pulse in a food processor until broken down into very small pieces or grate on the large holes of a box grater before sautéing. Alternatively, steam the whole florets for 10 minutes before blending with the other ingredients.

Per Serving (1¼ cups): Calories: 320; Total Fat: 25g; Protein: 15g; Carbohydrates: 10g; Fiber: 4g

Spinach and Shroom Scramble

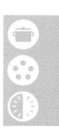

Vegetarian, Nut-Free
Serves 4 / Prep time: 5 minutes / **Cook time:** 10 minutes

Veggie scrambles are a fast and easy way to pack your first meal of the day with tons of nutrients. Lightly mixing the eggs into the mushrooms ensures they'll stay tender. Don't love mushrooms? Swap in chopped bell peppers, tomatoes, onions, or sliced olives instead. The healthy ingredients, ease of preparation, and great taste make this scramble a perfect Paleo breakfast.

3 tablespoons ghee or avocado oil, divided
4 cups sliced button mushrooms
½ teaspoon sea salt
¼ teaspoon freshly ground black pepper
8 large eggs
4 cups baby spinach

1. In a large pan, melt 2 tablespoons of the ghee over medium heat and then add the mushrooms, salt, and pepper. Cook, stirring occasionally, for 4 to 5 minutes, until the mushrooms soften and start to brown.

2. Add the remaining 1 tablespoon ghee to the pan and gently drop each egg on top of the mushrooms, spacing them evenly around the pan. Cook for 2 to 3 minutes, until the eggs start to set. With a spatula, lightly stir the whole mixture together, breaking all the egg yolks.

3. Add the spinach and, with a spatula, fold the mixture together until the spinach is wilted and all the ingredients are combined. Enjoy!

Switch It Up: For variety, use any type of leafy green, such as kale, chard, or collard greens, and any variety of mushroom, such as shiitake or baby bella mushrooms.

....

Per Serving (1 cup): Calories: 258; Total Fat: 20g; Protein: 20g; Carbohydrates: 4g; Fiber: 2g

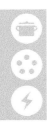

Meaty Breakfast Skillet

AIP, Egg-Free, Nut-Free
Serves 4 / Prep time: 5 minutes / **Cook time:** 5 minutes

When possible, choose grass-fed over conventionally raised beef. Why? Grass-fed meat contains higher levels of anti-inflammatory omega-3 fatty acids and fewer inflammatory omega-6s. Because grass-fed animals are never fed grain, they have less inflammation in their bodies and are less likely to get sick. This means they are rarely administered the antibiotics and hormones given to conventionally raised animals.

2 teaspoons
  avocado oil
1 pound ground beef,
  ground turkey, or
  ground pork
1 teaspoon Italian
  seasoning
½ teaspoon onion
  powder
¾ teaspoon sea salt
¼ teaspoon freshly
  ground black pepper
1 zucchini
4 cups baby spinach
2 cups berries

1. In a large pan, heat the oil over medium-high heat. Add the ground beef, Italian seasoning, onion powder, salt, and pepper and cook, stirring frequently, until the beef is almost browned, 4 to 5 minutes. With a spoon, remove all but 2 tablespoons of the rendered fat from the pan.

2. While the beef cooks, finely dice the zucchini.

3. Stir the zucchini and spinach into the pan and cook for 2 to 3 minutes, until the spinach has wilted and the zucchini is cooked to your liking.

4. Serve with ½ cup berries on the side of each serving.

Switch It Up: Crack 1 to 3 eggs into this recipe to pump up the protein. Make breakfast tacos by adding store-bought salsa and serving in Paleo Tortillas (page 160).

Per Serving (¾ cup beef and ½ cup berries): Calories: 217; Total Fat: 9g; Protein: 27g; Carbohydrates: 10g; Fiber: 5g

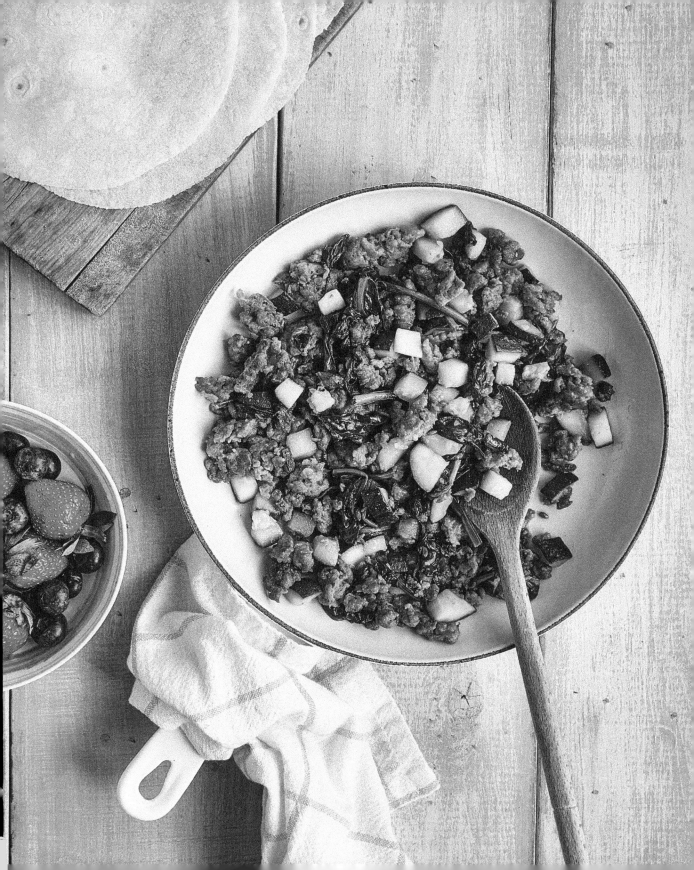

Almond Banana Pancakes with Blackberry Sauce

Vegetarian
Serves 4 / **Prep time:** 10 minutes / **Cook time:** 20 minutes

Almond flour contains more protein and fewer carbs than grain flours, so these pancakes will satisfy you longer while increasing your nutrient intake.

FOR THE BLACKBERRY SAUCE

1 cup blackberries, fresh or thawed frozen
¼ cup water

FOR THE PANCAKES

3 ripe bananas, peeled
4 large eggs
1 tablespoon pure vanilla extract
2 teaspoons freshly squeezed lemon juice (from ½ lemon)
1 cup almond flour
2 tablespoons tapioca flour
½ teaspoon baking soda
¼ teaspoon sea salt
Avocado oil, ghee, or coconut oil, for cooking

1. **Make the blackberry sauce:** In a small saucepan, combine the blackberries and water. Bring to a simmer over medium heat, then turn off the heat. Use an immersion blender to puree the sauce directly in the pan, or carefully transfer the sauce to a blender and puree. Set aside.

2. **Make the pancakes:** In a blender or food processor, puree the bananas, eggs, vanilla, and lemon juice. Add the almond flour, tapioca flour, baking soda, and salt. Blend until thoroughly mixed. Set aside.

3. In a large skillet over medium-low heat, heat enough oil to cover the bottom of the pan. Spoon 2 to 3 tablespoons of batter per pancake into the skillet to make 3- to 4-inch pancakes. Cook until bubbles appear on the surface, 1 to 2 minutes, then flip and cook for 1 to 2 minutes more on the second side. Watch the pancakes carefully—they quickly go from perfectly cooked to burned. Coat the pan with oil between batches as needed.

4. Enjoy the pancakes topped with blackberry sauce.

Switch It Up: Try berries in the spring, peaches in the summer, pears in the fall, and kiwis in the winter.

Per Serving (5 pancakes and 5 tablespoons sauce):
Calories: 319; Total Fat: 17g; Protein: 13g; Carbohydrates: 31g; Fiber: 5g

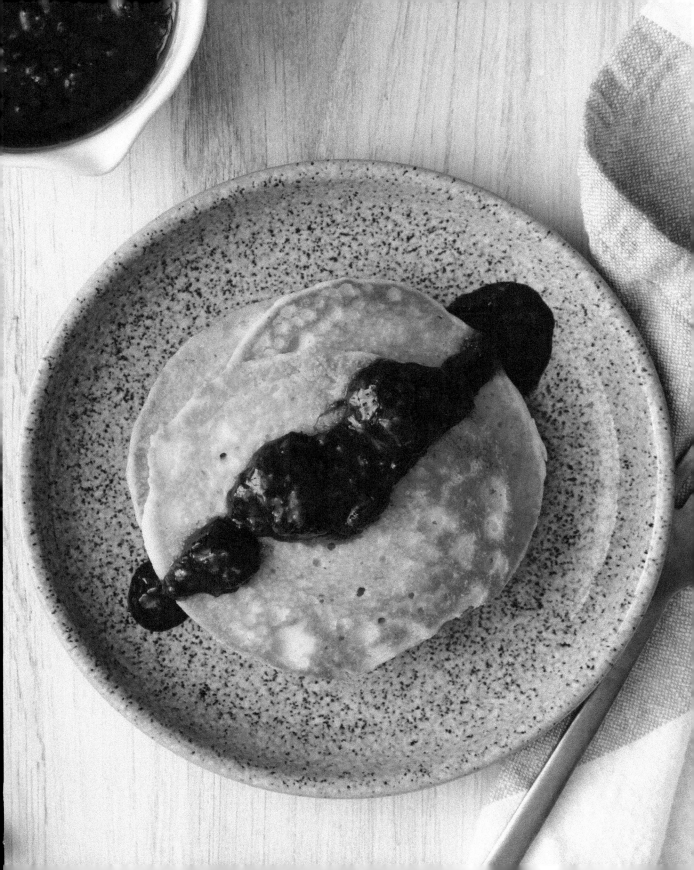

Good Day Green Smoothie

No-Cook, Egg-Free
Serves 2 / Prep time: 5 minutes

Smoothies are the perfect way to sneak nutritious greens into your diet every day. Dark green leafy veggies are a source of bioavailable nutrients including B vitamins, calcium, iron, magnesium, potassium, and fiber. This smoothie tastes so delicious, you won't even know it's chock-full of healthy greens!

2 cups stemmed kale leaves

2 cups green grapes, fresh or frozen

1 cup almond milk or coconut water

½ avocado

½ cup ice (if using fresh grapes)

¼ cup collagen powder or protein powder

1. In a blender, combine the kale, grapes, almond milk, avocado, ice (if using), and collagen powder. Puree until smooth.

2. Enjoy immediately for maximum nutrition. Refrigerate leftovers in an airtight container for up to 3 days. To serve leftovers, re-blend, adding ice as needed.

Technique Tip: Double the recipe and create not only a smoothie but also a healthy green dessert. Simply pour half the blended mixture into ice pop molds, then freeze for a future snack.

Per Serving (1½ cups): Calories: 257; Total Fat: 9g; Protein: 12g; Carbohydrates: 37g; Fiber: 7g

Berry Protein Muffins

Makes 12 muffins / Prep time: 10 minutes **/ Cook time:** 20 minutes

These berry muffins contain a healthy dose of protein from almond flour, eggs, and collagen which provide essential amino acids to help build muscle and burn fat. So, you can feel good about eating them!

3 large eggs
⅓ cup honey
⅓ cup coconut oil or ghee, melted
1 teaspoon pure vanilla extract
1½ cups almond flour
½ cup tapioca flour
½ cup collagen powder or protein powder
½ teaspoon baking soda
¼ teaspoon sea salt
1 cup fresh blueberries or berries of choice

1. Preheat the oven to 350°F. Line a 12-cup muffin tin with paper liners if you aren't using silicone baking cups.

2. In a food processor or blender, combine the eggs, honey, oil, and vanilla and process until combined. (Alternatively, mix by hand in a medium bowl using a large spoon.)

3. Add the almond flour, tapioca flour, collagen, baking soda, and salt to the wet ingredients and mix until thoroughly combined. Gently stir the blueberries into the batter by hand. Divide the batter evenly among the prepared muffin cups.

4. Bake for 20 minutes, then remove from the oven. Allow the muffins to cool in the pan for at least 10 minutes before transferring to the refrigerator to finish setting up before serving or storing.

Switch It Up: To add lemony flavor to this recipe, grate the zest from 1 to 2 lemons and stir it into the batter. Use a zester, Microplane, or the small holes of a box grater to shave the yellow zest off the lemon's bitter white pith.

Per Serving (3 muffins): Calories: 624; Total Fat: 40g; Protein: 22g; Carbohydrates: 51g; Fiber: 6g

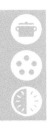

Grab-and-Go Egg Bites

Nut-Free
Serves 4 / Prep time: 10 minutes / **Cook time:** 20 minutes

These little pops of protein make it easy to stay the Paleo course on days when meal planning isn't a top priority. Chopped cauliflower, mushrooms, and even chopped leafy greens like spinach will work wonderfully. These egg bites freeze well, too, so make a double or triple batch to have a grab-and-go Paleo breakfast at the ready.

8 large eggs
7 ounces Canadian
   bacon or cooked ham
1 cup broccoli florets
1 medium bell pepper
½ teaspoon onion
   powder
¼ teaspoon sea salt
¼ teaspoon freshly
   ground black pepper

1. Preheat the oven to 350°F. Line a 12-cup muffin tin with paper if you are not using silicone baking cups.

2. In a large bowl, use a fork or a whisk to beat the eggs. Set aside. Chop the Canadian bacon, broccoli, and bell pepper into small pieces. Stir the bacon and vegetables into the eggs and add the onion powder, salt, and pepper.

3. Divide the egg mixture evenly among the prepared muffin cups, filling each about three-quarters full (the egg bites will rise during baking). Bake for 18 to 20 minutes, until the eggs are set. Remove from the oven and serve.

Appliance Tip: Silicone muffin cups eliminate the need for paper liners.

Per Serving (3 egg bites): Calories: 215; Total Fat: 12g; Protein: 23g; Carbohydrates: 3g; Fiber: 1g

Green Eggs and Ham Stir-Fry

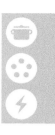

Nut-Free
Serves 2 / Prep time: 5 minutes **/ Cook time:** 5 minutes

We love green eggs and ham, and you will, too. It takes just a minute, a blender, some avocado, and some spinach to make your eggs all the more incredible. Stir-fried with tasty, salty ham, these green eggs make a great breakfast even Dr. Seuss would be proud of.

6 ounces cooked ham

4 teaspoons ghee or
   avocado oil, divided

4 large eggs

½ avocado

2 cups baby spinach,
   divided

¼ teaspoon sea salt

¼ teaspoon freshly
   ground black pepper

1. Cut the ham into large dice.

2. In a large pan, melt 2 teaspoons of the ghee over medium heat. Add the ham and cook until the ham starts to brown, 2 to 3 minutes.

3. While the ham cooks, in a blender, combine the eggs, avocado, 1 cup of the spinach, the salt, and pepper and blend until smooth.

4. Add the remaining 2 teaspoons ghee and 1 cup spinach to the pan with the ham and cook until the spinach has wilted, about 1 minute. Using a rubber spatula, scrape the egg mixture out of the blender into the pan, pouring it over the ham and spinach. Cook, stirring continuously, until the egg is scrambled to your liking. Enjoy!

Switch It Up: If you prefer your eggs a bit less green, skip the blender in step 3. Instead, add all the spinach to the pan with the ham in step 4. Beat the eggs, then pour them into the pan with the ham and spinach and season with the salt and pepper. Serve the avocado on the side.

Per Serving (1 cup): Calories: 401; Total Fat: 28g; Protein: 32g; Carbohydrates: 6g; Fiber: 3g

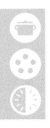

Sausage Frittata

Nut-Free
Serves 4 / Prep time: 10 minutes / **Cook time:** 20 minutes

Frittatas are baked egg dishes similar to omelets, and traditional frittata recipes often contain cheese. You won't miss the cheese in this super-satisfying Paleo frittata because it's chock-full of sausage, sweet potatoes, and greens.

1 large sweet potato
10 large eggs
⅓ cup full-fat coconut milk or almond milk
¼ teaspoon sea salt
¼ teaspoon freshly ground black pepper
2 teaspoons seasoning of choice, such as Italian seasoning, dried sage, thyme, etc. (optional)
2 tablespoons avocado oil, ghee, or bacon fat
8 ounces ground sausage
4 cups stemmed kale leaves

1. Preheat the oven to 350°F.

2. Chop the sweet potato into small dice or pulse in a food processor until chopped into small pieces.

3. In a medium bowl, whisk together the eggs, coconut milk, salt, pepper, and seasoning (if using).

4. In an oven-safe skillet, heat the oil over medium-high heat. Add the sweet potatoes and cook, stirring occasionally, until softened, about 5 minutes. Add the sausage and cook, stirring frequently, until the meat is browned, about 5 minutes. Add the kale and cook for 1 minute. Pour the egg mixture over the potatoes, sausage, and kale. Place the pan in the oven and bake for 15 to 20 minutes, until the eggs are set. Remove the frittata from the oven, cut into quarters, and enjoy.

Switch It Up: The kale crisps up nicely in this frittata, but you can use any variety of greens. Try spinach, collard greens, or chard.

....

Per Serving (¼ frittata): Calories: 479; Total Fat: 37g; Protein: 26g; Carbohydrates: 10g; Fiber: 2g

Nutty Paleo Cereal

Vegan, Egg-Free
Serves 4 / Prep time: 10 minutes **/ Cook time:** 10 minutes

Believe it or not, you can still enjoy cereal on the Paleo diet. Just swap out the grains and refined sugars for healthy ingredients like nuts, seeds, dried fruit, and coconut flakes, and you'll have a sweet, Paleo-worthy bowl. This recipe boasts the flavors and aromas of vanilla and cinnamon.

1 cup chopped almonds
½ cup chopped
  unsweetened dried
  apples
½ cup hulled sunflower
  seeds
2 tablespoons coconut
  oil, melted
2 teaspoons pure
  vanilla extract
1½ teaspoons ground
  cinnamon
¼ teaspoon sea salt
1½ cups fresh
  blueberries
1 cup unsweetened
  coconut flakes
Paleo-friendly milk,
  optional

1. Preheat the oven to 350°F.

2. In a medium bowl, stir together the almonds, apples, sunflower seeds, melted oil, vanilla, cinnamon, and salt.

3. Evenly spread the mixture in a baking sheet. Bake until it starts to brown, 10 to 12 minutes. Remove from the oven and stir in the berries and coconut flakes.

4. Enjoy the cereal on its own or top it with your favorite Paleo-friendly milk. Refrigerate leftovers in an airtight container at room temperature for up to 1 week.

Switch It Up: You can make this cereal nut-free by substituting pumpkin seeds, hemp seeds, or a combination for the almonds.

....

Per Serving (1 cup): Calories: 429; Total Fat: 31g; Protein: 10g; Carbohydrates: 26g; Fiber: 9g

Very Berry Smoothie

No-Cook, Egg-Free, Nut-Free
Serves 2 / Prep time: 5 minutes

Tastes like a milkshake but with none of the downsides! Berries are chock-full of antioxidants, vitamin C, and fiber, and cinnamon is loaded with antioxidants and anti-inflammatory properties. The boost of collagen helps repair bones, skin, muscles, tendons, and ligaments. This breakfast tastes like a dessert!

2 cups frozen berries (any type)
1 banana, peeled and frozen
¼ cup collagen powder or protein powder
1½ cups almond milk or coconut milk
½ teaspoon ground cinnamon

1. In a blender, combine the berries, banana, collagen, almond milk, and cinnamon. Puree until smooth.

2. Enjoy immediately for maximum nutrition. Refrigerate leftovers in an airtight container for up to 3 days. To serve leftovers, re-blend, adding ice as needed.

Ingredient Tip: Frozen berries and frozen banana add a nice thickness to smoothies. If you don't have frozen fruit, fresh berries and banana can be used—just add enough ice to achieve the desired consistency.

Per Serving (2 cups): Calories: 245; Total Fat: 3g; Protein: 23g; Carbohydrates: 39g; Fiber: 6g

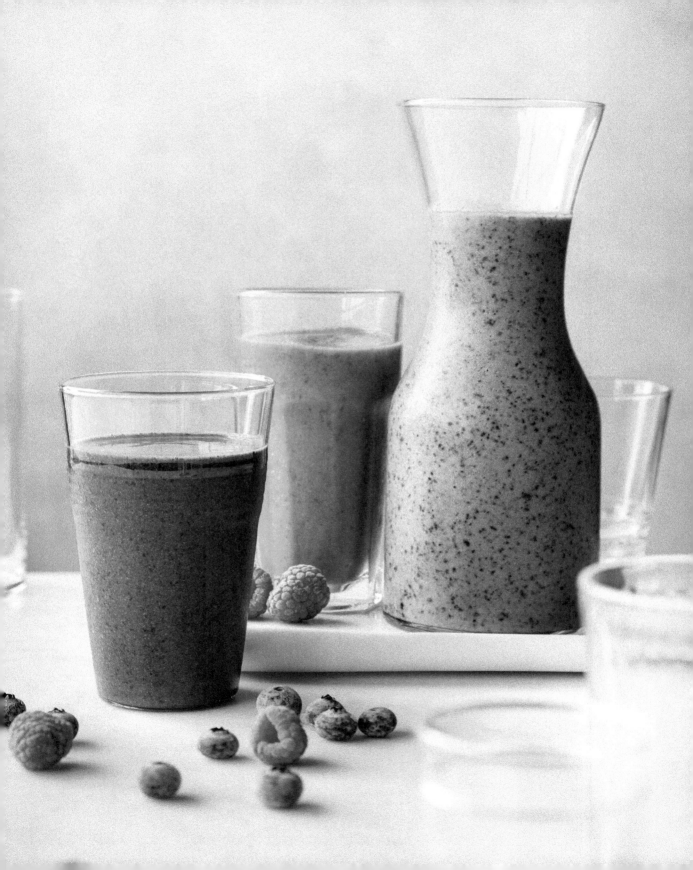

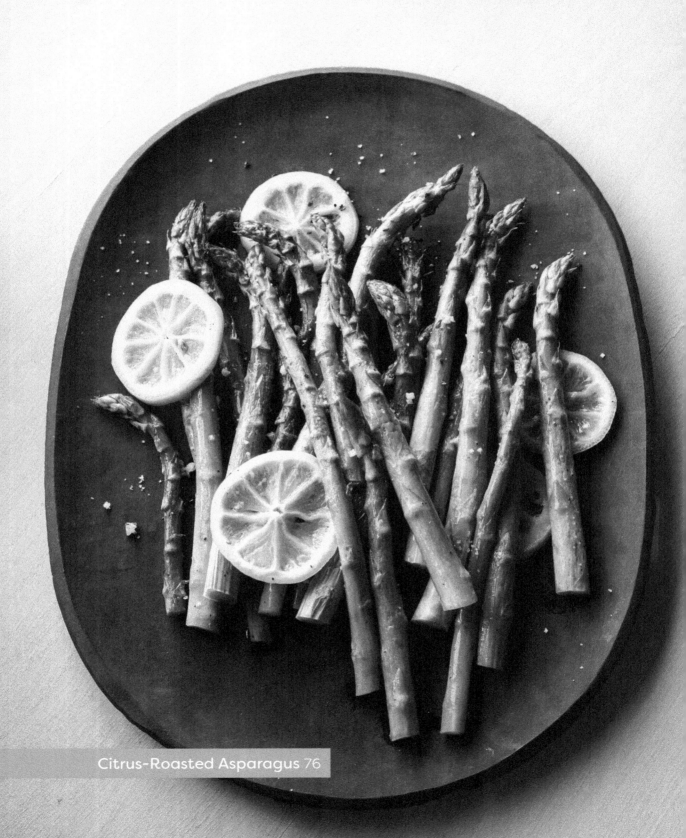

Citrus-Roasted Asparagus 76

CHAPTER 4

Vegetables and Side Dishes

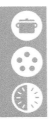

Zesty Zoodles

Vegan, Egg-Free, Nut-Free
Serves 4 / Prep time: 10 minutes / **Cook time:** 5 minutes

Have you been missing pasta? Zucchini noodles ("zoodles") are a grain-free, low-carb, Paleo-friendly version of traditional grain-based noodles. Cut to size from angel-hair thin to egg-noodle thick, zoodles are a great replacement for pasta in any recipe. Make your zoodles from green zucchini or yellow summer squash, or combine the two for "pasta" with pizzazz. If you'd like to add "cheese" to this dish, sprinkle some nutritional yeast over your cooked zoodles. These zoodles make a great side dish for Halibut with Basil Coconut Cream (page 92).

3 large zucchini

2 garlic cloves

2 tablespoons avocado oil

¼ teaspoon red pepper flakes, plus more if needed

¼ teaspoon sea salt

1. Use a regular vegetable peeler to slice thin, wide zoodles from the zucchini, stopping when you reach the seedy core; discard the cores or chop and refrigerate for another use. Finely chop the garlic.

2. In a large pan, heat the oil over medium heat. Add the garlic and red pepper flakes and cook until fragrant, about 30 seconds. Add the zoodles, salt, and more red pepper flakes, if needed, and cook for 2 to 3 minutes, until the zoodles start to soften.

Appliance Tip: To make zoodles of different sizes or shapes, use a mandoline, julienne peeler, or spiralizer.

Per Serving (½ cup): Calories: 93; Total Fat: 7g; Protein: 2g; Carbohydrates: 7g; Fiber: 2g

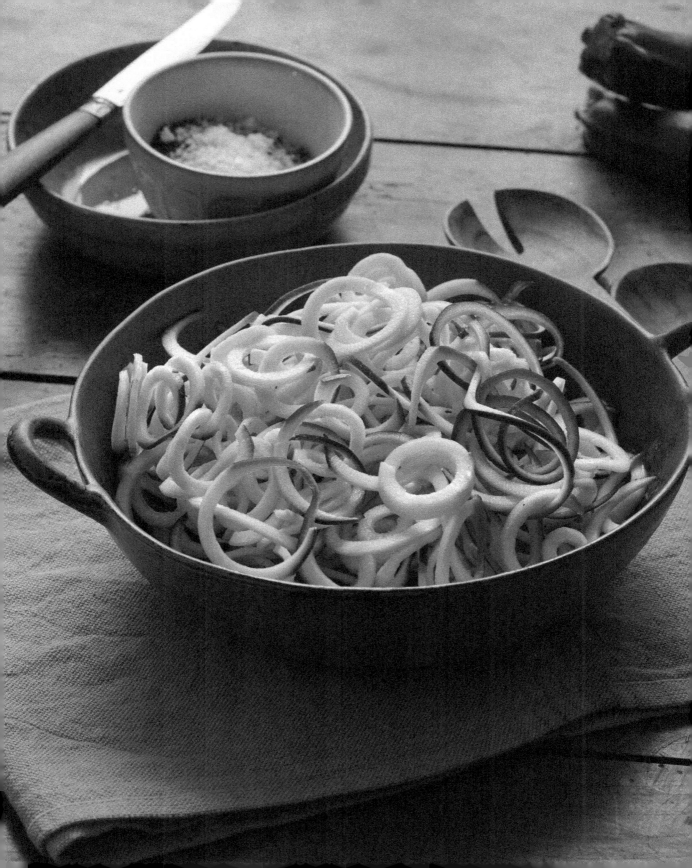

Sweet Potato Fries

Vegan, AIP, Egg-Free, Nut-Free
Serves 4 / Prep time: 5 minutes / **Cook time:** 15 minutes

Sweet potatoes are a carbohydrate staple for Paleo folks. Unlike white potatoes, sweet potatoes do not belong to the potentially inflammatory nightshade plant family. This makes them a perfect potato choice for those following the autoimmune protocol (AIP). One of our favorite ways to cook sweet potatoes is to cut them into fries and roast them. Serve these fries with Tomato Ketchup (page 164) or Paleo Ranch Dressing (page 166) on the side.

3 medium sweet
   potatoes
1 tablespoon
   avocado oil
1 teaspoon sea salt

1. Preheat the oven to 425°F.

2. Use a sharp knife to cut the sweet potatoes lengthwise into ½-inch-thick fries. Put the fries in a large bowl and toss with the oil and salt.

3. Arrange the fries in a single layer on a large baking sheet and bake for 15 to 20 minutes, until tender and browned to your liking. Remove from the oven and enjoy.

Switch It Up: Get out of your comfort zone and explore the range of colors, textures, and flavors of the sweet potato world. Instead of the typical orange-fleshed Jewel sweet potatoes, try creamy yellow Hannah sweet potatoes or Okinawan purple sweet potatoes.

Per Serving (2 cups): Calories: 115; Total Fat: 4g; Protein: 2g; Carbohydrates: 20g; Fiber: 3g

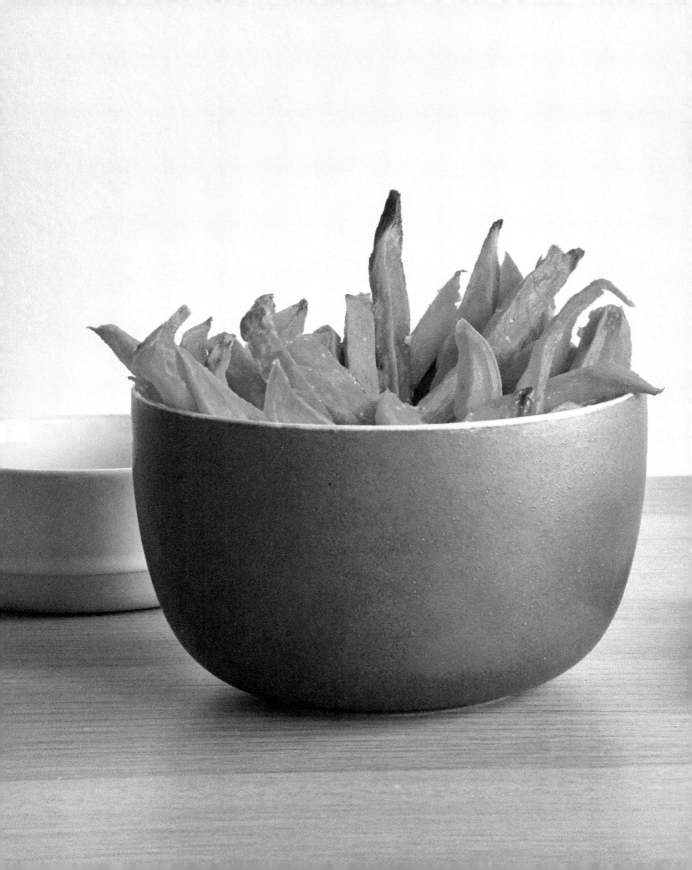

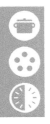

Roasted Brussels Sprouts

Vegan, Egg-Free, Nut-Free
Serves 4 / Prep time: 5 minutes / **Cook time:** 15 minutes

Originally cultivated in Brussels, Belgium, where they get their name, these splendid sprouts are enjoying their 15 minutes of culinary fame. Brussels sprouts can be cooked just about every which way: steamed, boiled, sautéed, baked. We love them roasted so they become crispy and develop a deep, delicious flavor. Brussels sprouts are also a cruciferous nutritional superstar, rich in disease-fighting plant compounds, as well as vitamins C and K. These Brussels sprouts make a great side dish for Savory Slow-Cooker Drumsticks (page 122).

4 cups Brussels sprouts

3 tablespoons avocado oil or ghee

½ teaspoon sea salt

¼ teaspoon garlic powder or onion powder

1. Preheat the oven to 400°F.

2. Trim the ends from the sprouts and remove any loose outer leaves. Slice in halves. In a large bowl, toss the sprouts with the oil, salt, and garlic powder to coat.

3. Transfer the sprouts to a baking sheet and roast for 15 minutes, until crispy and starting to char, tossing once halfway through the cooking time.

Technique Tip: We also love Brussels sprouts shredded and sautéed. Simply thinly slice them and cook in a skillet over medium-high heat in ghee or avocado oil with a pinch of sea salt until tender.

Per Serving (¾ cup): Calories: 128; Total Fat: 11g; Protein: 3g; Carbohydrates: 8g; Fiber: 3g

Garlicky Creamed Greens

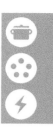

Vegan, Egg-Free, Nut-Free
Serves 4 / Prep time: 5 minutes / **Cook time:** 5 minutes

Toasted garlic melds with creamy coconut milk in this simple but flavorful Paleo rendition of creamed spinach. Spinach is a nutrient-dense superfood: it's a rich source of insoluble fiber, antioxidants, beta-carotene, vitamin C, vitamin K, folate, iron, and calcium. This recipe offers a delicious and simple way to get your daily dose of spinach. We've used baby spinach, but chopped mature spinach works just as well.

3 tablespoons coconut oil or ghee

6 garlic cloves, minced

16 cups baby spinach

⅔ cup full-fat coconut milk

¾ teaspoon sea salt

¾ teaspoon freshly ground black pepper

1. In a large skillet, heat the oil over medium heat. Add the garlic and cook, stirring, until it starts to turn golden, 1 to 2 minutes. Reduce the heat to low.

2. Add the spinach, coconut milk, salt, and pepper and stir to combine. Cook, stirring occasionally, for 2 to 3 minutes, until the spinach just starts to wilt.

3. Enjoy alongside your favorite protein.

Switch It Up: Any type of leafy green, such as chopped chard, kale, collards greens, and more, can be used in place of spinach in this recipe.

Per Serving (⅓ cup): Calories: 197; Total Fat: 19g; Protein: 4g; Carbohydrates: 7g; Fiber: 4g

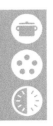

Roasted Radishes

Vegan, AIP, Egg-Free, Nut-Free
Serves 2 / Prep time: 5 minutes **/ Cook time:** 20 minutes

If you think you don't like radishes, this recipe will change your mind. Roasting is a unique and delicious way to prepare this spicy root vegetable. The high, dry heat initiates the chemical process of caramelization, which brings out the sweetness of the radishes that's otherwise masked by the peppery kick they're known for. Serve these roasted roots in place of potatoes for a low-carb and low-calorie side dish.

1 bunch radishes
   (about 10)
1 tablespoon
   avocado oil
½ teaspoon dried
   thyme
⅛ teaspoon sea salt,
   plus more if needed
⅛ teaspoon freshly
   ground black pepper
½ lemon, cut into
   wedges (optional)

1. Preheat the oven to 400°F.

2. Trim off the tops of the radishes, then halve the radishes lengthwise, cutting any larger radishes into quarters.

3. In a small bowl, mix together the oil, thyme, salt, and pepper. Toss the radishes in the dressing to coat.

4. Spread the radishes out on a baking sheet and roast until they are tender yet still firm in the center, 20 to 30 minutes.

5. Finish with a squeeze of lemon juice (if using) and additional salt, if desired.

Switch It Up: Transform this dish into roasted garlic radishes by adding 2 garlic cloves (minced) or ½ teaspoon garlic powder to the dressing in step 3.

Per Serving (5 radishes): Calories: 75; Total Fat: 7g; Protein: 1g; Carbohydrates: 3g; Fiber: 1g

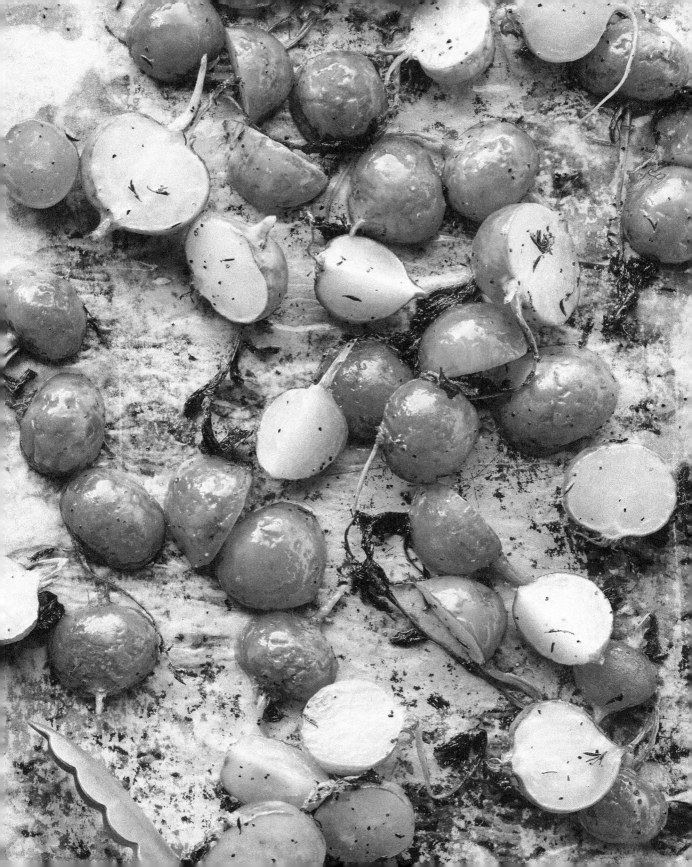

Simple Cauliflower Rice

Vegan, Egg-Free, Nut-Free
Serves 4 / Prep time: 5 minutes / **Cook time:** 10 minutes

For many, rice is a culinary essential, and to give it up is a Paleo deal breaker. This may sound optimistic, but we bet you'll love cauliflower rice so much that you won't miss the real thing at all. Cauliflower rice can be seasoned with an endless array of healthy fats, sauces, herbs, and add-ins, or served plain. No matter how you dress it up or down, it's a nutritious, delicious, and satisfying substitute for rice. Try it with Beef-tastic Tacos (page 127).

1 large head
   cauliflower, or 4 cups
   riced cauliflower (see
   tip on page 46)
1 to 3 teaspoons
   seasoning of choice
   (garlic powder, onion
   powder, dried parsley,
   etc.)
2 tablespoons
   avocado oil, ghee,
   or coconut oil
¼ teaspoon sea salt
¼ teaspoon freshly
   ground black pepper

1. If using a head of cauliflower, break it into florets and put in a food processor. Pulse several times, until the cauliflower resembles grains of rice. (Alternatively, finely dice the cauliflower by hand or grate it on the large holes of a box grater.) Transfer the riced cauliflower into a large bowl and toss with your seasoning of choice.

2. In a large pan, heat the oil over medium heat. Add the riced cauliflower to the pan, then season with the salt and pepper. Cook, stirring occasionally, for 10 minutes, or until the cauliflower is tender.

Ingredient Tip: You can save yourself precious prep time by purchasing fresh or frozen riced cauliflower in the produce or freezer section of your market.

Per Serving (1 cup): Calories: 96; Total Fat: 7g; Protein: 3g; Carbohydrates: 7g; Fiber: 3g

Sesame Ginger Slaw

No-Cook, Vegan, Egg-Free
Serves 4 / Prep time: 15 minutes

Most seed oils are unhealthy and not Paleo. However, unrefined sesame oil contains antioxidant lignans like sesamin, sesamol, and sesamolin, which have abundant health benefits. This Asian-inspired slaw features toasted sesame oil, which has a nuttier flavor than untoasted, but either can be used in this recipe. This slaw is fast to prepare in your food processor: use the shredding disc to slice the cabbage, then switch to the S-blade and pulse to chop the rest of the veggies.

½ head cabbage, shredded (8 cups)
1 bell pepper, diced
2 scallions, sliced
¼ cup chopped fresh cilantro
¼ cup coconut aminos
3 tablespoons toasted sesame oil
3 tablespoons apple cider vinegar
3 tablespoons almond butter
1 teaspoon minced garlic, or ¼ teaspoon garlic powder
2 teaspoons grated fresh ginger, or ¼ teaspoon ground ginger
¼ teaspoon sea salt
Sesame seeds, for garnish (optional)

1. Combine the cabbage, bell pepper, scallions, and cilantro in a large bowl.

2. In a blender, combine the coconut aminos, sesame oil, vinegar, almond butter, garlic, ginger, and salt and blend until well combined. (Alternatively, mix by hand in a small bowl.)

3. Add the dressing to the veggies and use tongs or your hands to mix.

4. Garnish with sesame seeds, if desired, and serve alongside your favorite protein.

Technique Tip: Prep this slaw in advance to save time at mealtime. Mix the dressing ingredients in a large bowl. Place the prepped veggies in the bowl over the dressing, but do not mix until you are ready to serve.

Per Serving (2 cups): Calories: 240; Total Fat: 18g; Protein: 5g; Carbohydrates: 17g; Fiber: 6g

Cauliflower Mash

Vegetarian, Egg-Free
Serves 4 / Prep time: 5 minutes / **Cook time:** 10 minutes

Cauliflower is magical; it can be cooked in myriad ways and transformed into just about any of your old conventional food favorites. In this recipe, we conjure up the silkiest, smoothest, tastiest mash you've ever eaten. Of course, you can eat mashed potatoes on the Paleo diet, but this recipe has the advantage of being low-carb and full of cruciferous-veggie nutrients like sulfur-containing antioxidants.

1 large head
   cauliflower, broken
   into florets, or 4 cups
   riced cauliflower
   (see tip on page 46)
   plus 1 additional
   tablespoon ghee or
   coconut oil
¼ cup almond milk or
   full-fat coconut milk
3 tablespoons ghee or
   coconut oil
½ teaspoon sea salt
¼ teaspoon freshly
   ground black pepper
¼ teaspoon garlic
   powder (optional)

1. Fill a saucepan with ¼ to ½ inch of water and set a steamer basket inside. Bring the water to a simmer, then add the cauliflower, cover, and steam until tender, about 10 minutes. (Alternatively, if you are using riced cauliflower, cook it in a large pan over medium heat in 1 tablespoon ghee or coconut oil until tender, about 10 minutes.)

2. Using a slotted spoon, carefully transfer the cauliflower to a blender. Add the almond milk, ghee, salt, pepper, and garlic powder (if using) and puree until smooth. (Alternatively, drain the cauliflower and return it to the pot, then add the remaining ingredients and use a potato masher or large fork to mash.)

Appliance Tip: To steam the cauliflower florets or riced cauliflower in the microwave in step 1, put the cauliflower in a microwave-safe bowl with 3 tablespoons water, cover, and microwave for 3 to 4 minutes, until soft.

·······································

Per Serving (½ cup): Calories: 133; Total Fat: 11g; Protein: 3g; Carbohydrates: 7g; Fiber: 3g

Root Vegetable Puree

Egg-Free, Nut-Free
Serves 4 / Prep time: 5 minutes / **Cook time:** 20 minutes

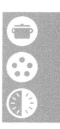

This silky puree has the texture of mashed potatoes with the sweetness and added health benefits of root vegetables. Carrots and parsnips are close root vegetable cousins, the only visual difference being the parsnips' ivory color. Because you're blending these root veggies into a puree, there's no need to peel them. By leaving the skins on, you'll save on prep time and provide yourself with extra nutrition.

4 garlic cloves
1 pound parsnips
  (4 medium), scrubbed
1 pound carrots
  (5 medium), scrubbed
2 tablespoons coconut
  oil or ghee
½ cup chicken broth or
  bone broth
½ cup water
1½ teaspoons sea salt
½ teaspoon freshly
  ground black pepper

1. Mince the garlic and coarsely chop the parsnips and carrots.

2. In a large pot, melt the coconut oil over medium heat. Add the garlic and cook, stirring continuously, until fragrant, about 1 minute.

3. Add the parsnips, carrots, broth, water, salt, and pepper to the pot. Bring to a boil. Reduce the heat to low, cover, and simmer for 20 minutes, or until the vegetables are soft enough to easily pierce with a fork.

4. Using an immersion blender, puree the mixture directly in the pot until smooth and well combined. (Alternatively, carefully transfer the mixture to a blender or food processor and puree.)

Switch It Up: Feel free to mix and match root veggies. Try substituting sweet potatoes for the carrots or turnips for the parsnips. Toss in a red beet to add vibrant color to your side dish.

Per Serving (½ cup): Calories: 207; Total Fat: 8g; Protein: 3g; Carbohydrates: 32g; Fiber: 9g

Best Balsamic Beets

Vegan, AIP, Egg-Free, Nut-Free
Serves 4 / Prep time: 5 minutes / **Cook time:** 45 minutes

Did you know that beets can improve athletic performance? They contain a high concentration of dietary nitrates that relax blood vessels and can lower blood pressure. What's more, beets get their beautiful ruby color from betalain pigments, which are known to have anti-inflammatory properties.

6 medium beets
2 tablespoons
  avocado oil
½ teaspoon sea salt
½ cup balsamic vinegar

1. Preheat the oven to 400°F. Line a rimmed baking sheet with parchment paper. Set aside.

2. Trim the beets (save the beet greens for a salad or sauté—they're delicious!) and cut them into 1-inch cubes. Combine in a bowl with the oil and salt and toss to coat.

3. Spread the beets out on a baking sheet and bake for 45 to 60 minutes, until tender when pierced with a fork.

4. While the beets cook, in a small pot, bring the vinegar to a simmer over low heat and cook until it reduces by one-third to half and thickens enough to coat the back of a spoon, about 10 minutes. Remove from the heat; the vinegar will continue to thicken a bit as it cools.

5. Drizzle the beets with the balsamic reduction and serve.

Technique Tip: If you overcook the vinegar, it will harden up. When this happens, add a couple of table-spoons of water and reheat until it is liquid again.

....

Per Serving (1 cup beets with glaze): Calories: 132; Total Fat: 7g; Protein: 2g; Carbohydrates: 18g; Fiber: 3g

Super Egg Salad

Vegetarian, Nut-Free
Serves 4 / Prep time: 10 minutes **/ Cook time:** 13 minutes

This picnic-perfect powerhouse takes typical egg salad to the next level. Cool spinach collides with crunchy sunflower seeds to add crave-worthy texture, flavor, and nutrition to this quick and easy salad. Crumble crispy bacon on top to make this egg salad even more super.

8 large eggs
⅓ cup Paleo
   Mayonnaise
   (page 163)
1 tablespoon Dijon
   mustard
1 tablespoon freshly
   squeezed lemon juice
   (from ½ lemon)
½ teaspoon dried dill
¼ teaspoon sea salt
¼ teaspoon freshly
   ground black pepper
⅛ teaspoon paprika
2 cups baby spinach
1 celery stalk
¼ red onion
¼ cup roasted
   sunflower seeds

1. Place a steamer basket in a medium pot and add enough water to reach the bottom of the basket. Cover and bring to a boil over high heat. Add the eggs, cover, and steam for 13 minutes. Transfer the eggs to an ice bath until cool.

2. While the eggs are cooking and cooling, in a small bowl, combine the mayonnaise, mustard, lemon juice, dill, salt, pepper, and paprika. Set aside.

3. Chop the spinach leaves and mince the celery and onion.

4. Peel the hard-boiled eggs, then chop them into small pieces and put them in a large bowl. Add the sauce, veggies, and sunflower seeds and gently mix until combined.

Switch It Up: Love pickles? Add ¼ cup chopped pickles or a splash of pickle juice to the sauce. Like it hot? Add a pinch of cayenne pepper.

Per Serving (¾ cup): Calories: 302; Total Fat: 26g; Protein: 14g; Carbohydrates: 3g; Fiber: 2g

Citrus-Roasted Asparagus

Vegan, AIP, Egg-Free, Nut-Free
Serves 4 / Prep time: 5 minutes **/ Cook time:** 20 minutes

Asparagus is low in calories but rich in nutrients like fiber, iron, B complex vitamins, and vitamins K, A, and C, and contains diuretic, anti-inflammatory, and antioxidant properties. This recipe is versatile, and any type of citrus can be used. Try subbing in an orange for the lemon and 2 tablespoons minced shallot for the garlic.

1 pound asparagus
   spears (20 to
   30 medium)
½ lemon
4 garlic cloves
1 tablespoon
   extra-virgin olive oil
1 teaspoon dried thyme
¼ teaspoon sea salt
⅛ teaspoon freshly
   ground black pepper

1. Adjust an oven rack to the uppermost position and preheat the oven to 400°F. Line a large baking sheet with parchment paper.

2. Trim the tough ends off the asparagus spears. Zest and juice the lemon half to yield 1 teaspoon zest and 1 tablespoon juice. (If you don't have a zester, use the small holes of a box grater.) Mince the garlic.

3. In a small bowl, whisk together the lemon juice, olive oil, thyme, salt, and pepper.

4. Arrange the asparagus in a row on the prepared baking sheet. Pour over the dressing and use your hands to thoroughly coat the spears. Sprinkle with the lemon zest and garlic. Place the baking sheet on the top rack in the oven and roast for 10 minutes, then shake the pan or use tongs to turn the spears. Roast for 10 minutes more, or until the asparagus is tender.

Ingredient Tip: Thicker asparagus spears withstand dry oven heat better than thin ones.

....

Per Serving (5 spears): Calories: 59; Total Fat: 4g; Protein: 3g; Carbohydrates: 6g; Fiber: 3g

Supergreen Salad with Raspberry Dressing

No-Cook, Vegan, Egg-Free
Serves 4 / Prep time: 10 minutes

This salad is brimming with superfoods to recharge your health while tasting fantastic. In addition to fiber, vitamins, and minerals, it provides a stunning base for the flavorful, antioxidant-rich raspberry vinaigrette. It's a blank canvas for any protein you want to add, such as shredded rotisserie chicken or bacon crumbles.

FOR THE DRESSING

¾ cup extra-virgin olive oil
⅓ cup raspberries
¼ cup balsamic vinegar
1 garlic clove
1 teaspoon Dijon mustard
¼ teaspoon sea salt
⅛ teaspoon freshly ground black pepper

FOR THE SALAD

1 large cucumber
2 cups broccoli florets
1 Granny Smith apple
4 cups baby kale
4 cups baby spinach
4 cups arugula
½ cup chopped walnuts

1. **Make the dressing:** In a blender or food processor, combine the oil, raspberries, vinegar, garlic, mustard, salt, and pepper. Puree until well combined and emulsified, then set aside.

2. **Make the salad:** Peel the cucumber; chop the cucumber and broccoli into bite-size pieces and combine in a large bowl. Core and thinly slice the apple. Add the apple, kale, spinach, arugula, and walnuts to the bowl.

3. When you are ready to serve, pour half the dressing over the salad and toss to coat. Store the leftover dressing in an airtight container in the refrigerator for up to 1 week.

Love Your Leftovers: The leftover raspberry vinaigrette makes a great dip for cut-up veggies, like carrots or radishes, and an excellent dressing for deli wraps.

Per Serving (3½ cups salad with dressing): Calories: 357; Total Fat: 29g; Protein: 6g; Carbohydrates: 19g; Fiber: 7g

Puree of Pumpkin Soup

Egg-Free, Nut-Free
Serves 4 / Prep time: 5 minutes **/ Cook time:** 5 minutes

This silky pumpkin soup is inspired by warming fall flavors. You can make it vegan by using vegetable broth, or swap in Homemade Bone Broth (page 168) for its gut-healing benefits. Blend the ingredients in advance for a simple heat-and-eat meal. Stir in a tablespoon of maple syrup at the end for a real treat!

2 (15-ounce) cans pure pumpkin puree

2 cups chicken broth

1 cup full-fat coconut milk

2 teaspoons onion powder

1 teaspoon sea salt

1 teaspoon garlic powder

½ teaspoon ground cinnamon

½ teaspoon ground ginger

¼ teaspoon freshly ground black pepper

¼ cup pumpkin seeds (optional)

¼ cup unsweetened coconut flakes (optional)

1. In a blender, combine the pumpkin, broth, coconut milk, onion powder, salt, garlic powder, cinnamon, ginger, and pepper and puree. (Alternatively, stir together the ingredients in a large bowl until well combined.) Pour the mixture into a medium soup pot.

2. Bring the soup to a simmer over medium-high heat, then reduce the heat to medium-low and simmer for 5 minutes.

3. Ladle into bowls, garnish with the pumpkin seeds and coconut flakes, if desired, and serve.

Ingredient Tip: Make your own pumpkin puree! Use a paring knife to pierce the skin of a small baking pumpkin several times. Place on a baking sheet and bake at 375°F for 45 to 60 minutes, until the flesh is easily pierced with a fork. Cut the pumpkin in half and scoop out the seeds (save them to roast later and enjoy as a snack). Scoop the pumpkin flesh into a bowl (discard the skin) and mash with a fork or puree in a food processor or blender.

Per Serving (1¾ cups): Calories: 192; Total Fat: 13g; Protein: 3g; Carbohydrates: 20g; Fiber: 5g

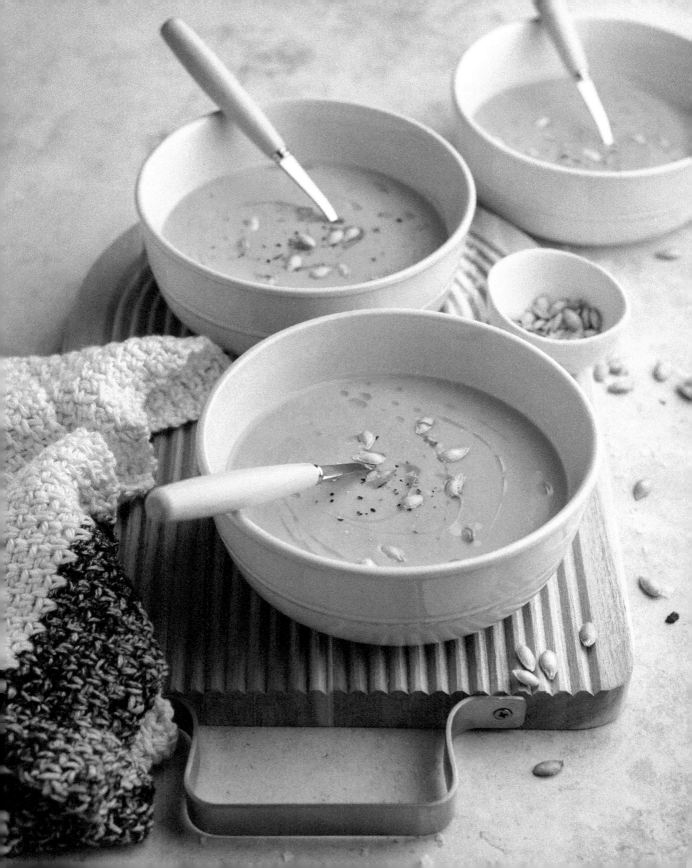

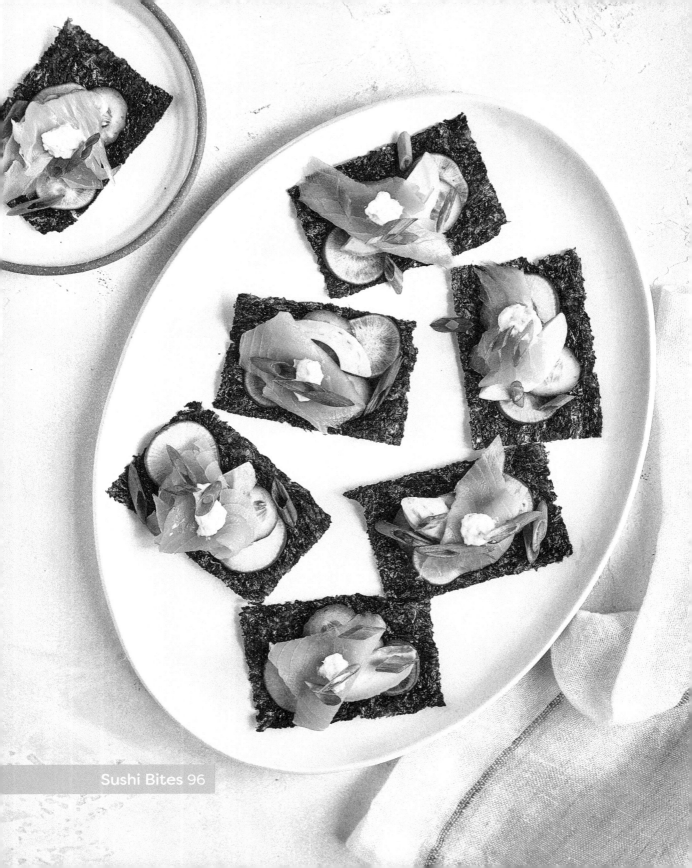

CHAPTER 5

Seafood

Easy Tuna Salad

No-Cook, Nut-Free
Serves 2 / Prep time: 10 minutes

Tuna is packed with high-quality muscle-building protein, vitamins, minerals, and anti-inflammatory omega-3 fatty acids. We've used canned tuna in this recipe because it's a minimally processed Paleo-friendly packaged food that makes the diet easy to stick to. This salad is chock-full of crunchy veggies and spiked with flavorful herbs. You can use store-bought Paleo-friendly mayonnaise or make your own (see page 163).

2 (5-ounce) cans tuna, drained

⅓ cup Paleo mayonnaise

1 small celery stalk, diced

½ small red onion, diced

3 tablespoons chopped fresh parsley

½ teaspoon dried dill

¼ teaspoon sea salt

¼ teaspoon freshly ground black pepper

4 cups mixed greens

1. Put the tuna in a large bowl. Add the mayo and mash with a fork until there are no large chunks.

2. Add the celery, onion, parsley, dill, salt, and pepper. Mix until combined.

3. Divide the mixed greens between two salad bowls or plates and top evenly with the tuna salad.

Smart Shopping: Our favorite brands of canned tuna are Safe Catch and Wild Planet, which source sustainably caught seafood.

Per Serving (¾ cup): Calories: 372; Total Fat: 27g; Protein: 25g; Carbohydrates: 5g; Fiber: 2g

Prosciutto Scallops

AIP, Egg-Free, Nut-Free
Serves 4 / Prep time: 5 minutes / **Cook time:** 10 minutes

Serve these scallops over Root Vegetable Puree (page 73) for a healthy and filling meal.

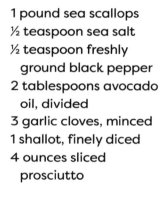

1 pound sea scallops
½ teaspoon sea salt
½ teaspoon freshly ground black pepper
2 tablespoons avocado oil, divided
3 garlic cloves, minced
1 shallot, finely diced
4 ounces sliced prosciutto

1. Preheat the broiler. Line a baking sheet with parchment paper.

2. Use paper towels to pat the scallops dry. Season with salt and pepper on both sides. Set aside.

3. In a medium skillet, heat 1 tablespoon of oil over medium heat. When hot, add the garlic and shallot and sauté until soft, 2 to 3 minutes. Remove and set aside.

4. In the same skillet, increase the heat to medium-high. Add up to 1 tablespoon of the remaining oil to coat the bottom of the pan, as needed. When pan is hot, sear the scallops for approximately 30 seconds per side. Transfer to the prepared baking sheet.

5. Wrap the prosciutto around the short sides of each scallop, leaving the flat sides exposed. Top each scallop with a dollop of the garlic and shallot mixture.

6. Broil the scallops until just cooked through, about 5 minutes. Enjoy!

Smart Shopping: No prosciutto on hand? Cook bacon until almost crispy but still bendable. Wrap it around the scallops prior to broiling.

....

Per Serving (4 ounces): Calories: 195; Total Fat: 10g; Protein: 20g; Carbohydrates: 7g; Fiber: 0g

Fish 'n' Fries

AIP, Egg-Free, Nut-Free
Serves 2 / Prep time: 15 minutes / **Cook time:** 30 minutes

Even if you aren't a seafood fan, it's hard not to love these delicious, crispy fish sticks, especially because they're so easy to make. Served with garlic-turmeric parsnip fries on the side, this healthy meal will quickly become one of your go-to favorites. Feel free to use any type of white-fleshed fish, such as cod, halibut, rockfish, or snapper, and serve the fries with Tomato Ketchup (page 164) for dipping, if you like.

FOR THE FRIES

3 parsnips

2 tablespoons tapioca flour or arrowroot flour

2 teaspoons garlic powder

1 teaspoon ground turmeric

1 teaspoon sea salt

½ teaspoon freshly ground black pepper

2 tablespoons avocado oil

1. Preheat the oven to 450°F. Line a baking sheet with parchment paper.

2. **Make the fries:** Peel and trim the parsnips, then cut them into sticks about 3 inches long and ½ inch thick. Set aside.

3. In a small bowl, combine the tapioca flour, garlic powder, turmeric, salt, and pepper. Pour the oil into a large bowl, then add the parsnips and toss to coat. Add the spice mixture and toss to coat.

4. Spread the parsnips out on the prepared baking sheet. Roast for 15 minutes, until they begin to brown at their edges, then flip and roast for 15 minutes more, or until tender.

5. **Make the fish:** In a small bowl, mix the tapioca flour, dill, salt, and pepper.

FOR THE FISH

⅓ cup tapioca flour or arrowroot flour

1 teaspoon dried dill

½ teaspoon sea salt

½ teaspoon freshly ground black pepper

1 pound boneless, skinless white-fleshed fish

3 tablespoons avocado oil

6. Pat the fish dry with a paper towel and cut it into roughly 1-by-3-inch strips. Roll the fish sticks in the batter to coat completely.

7. In a large skillet, heat the avocado oil over medium heat. When the oil is hot, carefully lay the fish sticks in the pan and fry for 4 to 5 minutes, then flip and fry for 3 to 4 minutes more, until golden brown.

8. Enjoy the fish sticks with the parsnip fries on the side.

Switch It Up: This recipe can be prepared with almond flour instead of tapioca flour. For the fries, simply exclude the tapioca flour. For the fish, beat an egg white in a shallow bowl. In a second shallow bowl, stir together ½ cup almond flour, ½ teaspoon dried dill, ¼ teaspoon salt, and ¼ teaspoon pepper. Dip the fish strips in the egg, then dredge in the almond flour to coat before frying.

Per Serving (5 fish sticks and about 20 fries): Calories: 644; Total Fat: 23g; Protein: 40g; Carbohydrates: 68g; Fiber: 14g

Red Curry Cod

Egg-Free, Nut-Free
Serves 4 / Prep time: 10 minutes / **Cook time:** 15 minutes

Red curry paste is a staple of Thai cuisine. It's a favorite ingredient in the Paleo cook's repertoire due to its versatility. In this recipe, red curry's smoky, slightly spicy essence infuses coconut milk with divine flavor. Kale adds vitamins, minerals, fiber, and color, and cod provides tender and flaky high-quality protein. Serve in a bowl on top of Simple Cauliflower Rice (page 70), if desired.

2½ cups chicken broth
1 (13.5-ounce) can full-fat coconut milk
5 tablespoons red curry paste
¼ teaspoon sea salt
¼ teaspoon freshly ground black pepper
1 bunch kale
1½ pounds skinless cod
½ cup chopped fresh cilantro, for garnish

1. In a large pot, combine the broth, coconut milk, curry paste, salt, and pepper. Bring to a simmer over medium heat, then cook for 5 minutes, stirring occasionally.

2. Remove the tough stems from the kale leaves and tear the leaves into bite-size pieces. Add the kale to the pot. Cover and simmer for 5 minutes, until the kale starts to wilt.

3. While the kale cooks, cut the cod into 1-inch pieces. When the kale has begun to wilt, add the cod to the pot and simmer, uncovered, for 4 to 5 minutes, until the fish is fully cooked.

4. Garnish with the cilantro and enjoy.

Smart Shopping: Thai Kitchen brand curry pastes are a Paleo-friendly favorite available in most major supermarkets and online. This recipe is also delicious using Thai Kitchen's green curry paste in place of the red variety.

....

Per Serving (1½ cups): Calories: 383; Total Fat: 24g; Protein: 35g; Carbohydrates: 12g; Fiber: 5g

Baked Salmon Cakes

Nut-Free
Serves 4 / Prep time: 10 minutes / **Cook time:** 20 minutes

A great source of high-quality protein, salmon provides the most omega-3 fatty acids of any fish, along with a host of vitamins and minerals. Farmed salmon is often exposed to environmental pollutants that wild salmon is not, so go wild when you can! Enjoy these salmon cakes alongside a leafy green salad, such as our Supergreen Salad with Raspberry Dressing (page 77).

1 small red onion

4 scallions

4 garlic cloves

2 (14-ounce) cans salmon

2 large eggs

¼ cup Paleo mayonnaise

2 tablespoons chopped fresh parsley, or 2 teaspoons dried

4 teaspoons Dijon mustard

2 teaspoons coconut flour

½ teaspoon sea salt

½ teaspoon freshly ground black pepper

1. Preheat the oven to 350°F. Line a 12-cup muffin tin with paper liners if not using silicone baking cups.

2. Finely chop the onion and the scallions, and mince the garlic. Set aside.

3. In a medium bowl, combine the onion, scallions, garlic, salmon, eggs, mayonnaise, parsley, mustard, coconut flour, salt, and pepper and stir until well mixed. Divide the mixture evenly among the prepared muffin cups.

4. Bake the salmon cakes for 20 to 25 minutes, until a toothpick inserted into the center comes out clean. Transfer the cakes to a wire rack to cool before serving.

Serving Tip: Serve cakes dolloped with lemon-dill mayo: Mix 1 cup mayonnaise, 1 tablespoon dried dill, and the zest and juice of 1 lemon.

Per Serving (3 cakes): Calories: 443; Total Fat: 22g; Protein: 48g; Carbohydrates: 7g; Fiber: 2g

Shrimp Scampi with Zoodles

Egg-Free, Nut-Free
Serves 4 / Prep time: 10 minutes **/ Cook time:** 10 minutes

This healthy shrimp scampi recipe has shrimp in a garlicky ghee scampi sauce with a hint of lemon and white wine, for a light and refreshing meal that's ready in only 20 minutes. You can use either dry white wine or broth (vegetable, chicken, or bone broth) in this recipe. Low-carb zucchini noodles (known as "zoodles") replace linguine in this good-for-you version.

4 medium zucchini

½ lemon

2 tablespoons ghee or extra-virgin olive oil

3 tablespoons extra-virgin olive oil, divided

1 small onion, diced

4 garlic cloves, minced

⅓ cup chicken broth or dry white wine

½ teaspoon sea salt

½ teaspoon freshly ground black pepper

¼ teaspoon red pepper flakes (optional)

1½ pounds raw large shrimp, peeled and deveined

⅓ cup finely chopped fresh parsley

1. Use a vegetable peeler or spiralizer to create noodles from the zucchini. Set aside.

2. Zest and juice the lemon to yield ½ teaspoon zest and 1 tablespoon juice. Set aside.

3. In a large skillet, melt the ghee with 2 tablespoons of oil over medium-high heat. Add the onion and garlic and cook, stirring, until fragrant, about 1 minute. Add the broth, salt, black pepper, and red pepper flakes (if using). Bring to a simmer, then cook for 2 minutes to reduce the broth.

4. Add the shrimp to the skillet and cook for 2 to 3 minutes per side, until they just turn pink. Stir in the lemon zest, lemon juice, and parsley. Remove the shrimp from the skillet and set aside.

5. In the same skillet, heat the remaining 1 tablespoon oil over medium-high heat. Add the zucchini noodles and cook, stirring frequently, until al dente, about 2 minutes.

6. Return the shrimp mixture to the pan with the zoodles and toss to combine, then serve.

....

Per Serving (6 ounces shrimp and 1 cup zoodles): Calories: 333; Total Fat: 20g; Protein: 24g; Carbohydrates: 8g; Fiber: 1g

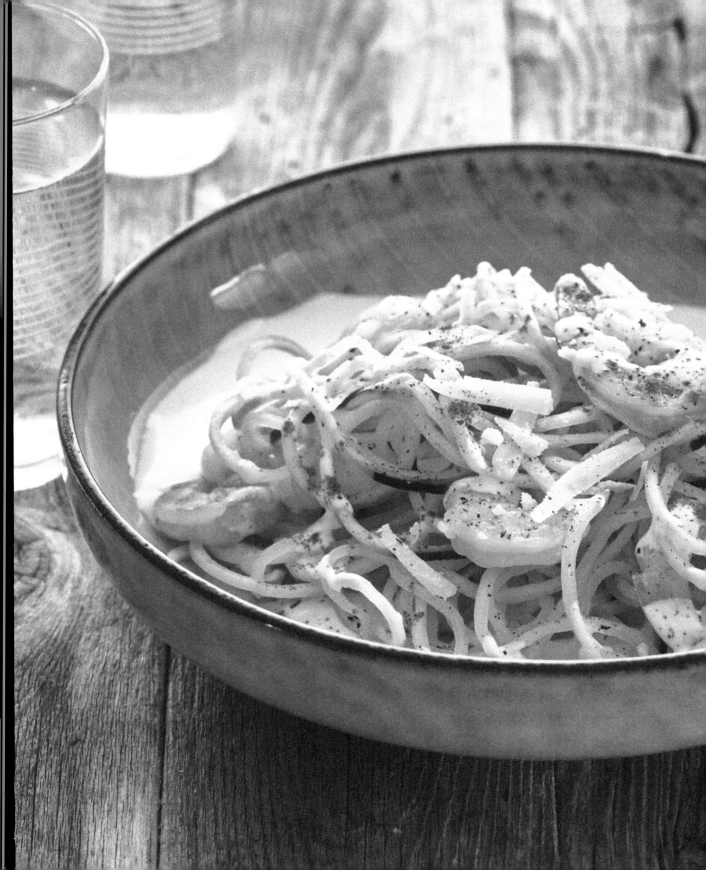

Fiery Chipotle Salmon with Salsa Salad

Egg-Free, Nut-Free
Serves 4 / Prep time: 10 minutes / **Cook time:** 15 minutes

Here chipotle salmon goes head-to-head with a snappy salsa, delivering bold and noteworthy flavors. Not a fan of chipotle? Swap in lemon pepper, dried dill, or chili powder instead.

FOR THE SALMON

1 tablespoon
   avocado oil
1 teaspoon ground
   chipotle chile
¾ teaspoon sea salt
½ teaspoon freshly
   ground black pepper
1½ pounds salmon

FOR THE SALSA SALAD

6 Roma (plum)
   tomatoes
1 medium avocado
1 small red onion
¾ cup chopped fresh
   cilantro
1 jalapeño (optional)
2 tablespoons freshly
   squeezed lime juice
   (from 1 lime)
1½ tablespoons
   extra-virgin olive oil
½ teaspoon sea salt
4 cups chopped
   romaine lettuce

1. **Make the salmon:** Preheat the oven to 375°F. Line a rimmed baking sheet with parchment paper.

2. In a small bowl, mix the avocado oil, chipotle, salt, and pepper.

3. Place the salmon on the prepared baking sheet, skin-side down, and rub the flesh side with the spice blend to cover.

4. Bake the salmon for 15 to 20 minutes, until it flakes easily with a fork.

5. **Make the salsa salad:** Chop the tomatoes, avocado, onion, cilantro, and jalapeño (if using). Combine in a large bowl, add the lime juice, oil, and salt, and mix.

6. Divide the lettuce among four plates and top evenly with the salsa. Enjoy the salmon alongside.

Technique Tip: To cook the salmon on the stovetop, place it flesh-side down in an oiled skillet. Cook over medium-high heat for 2 to 3 minutes, then flip, reduce the heat to low, and cook for 5 to 10 minutes more, until the salmon flakes easily with a fork.

Per Serving (6 ounces salmon plus salsa salad): Calories: 476; Total Fat: 30g; Protein: 38g; Carbohydrates: 17g; Fiber: 5g

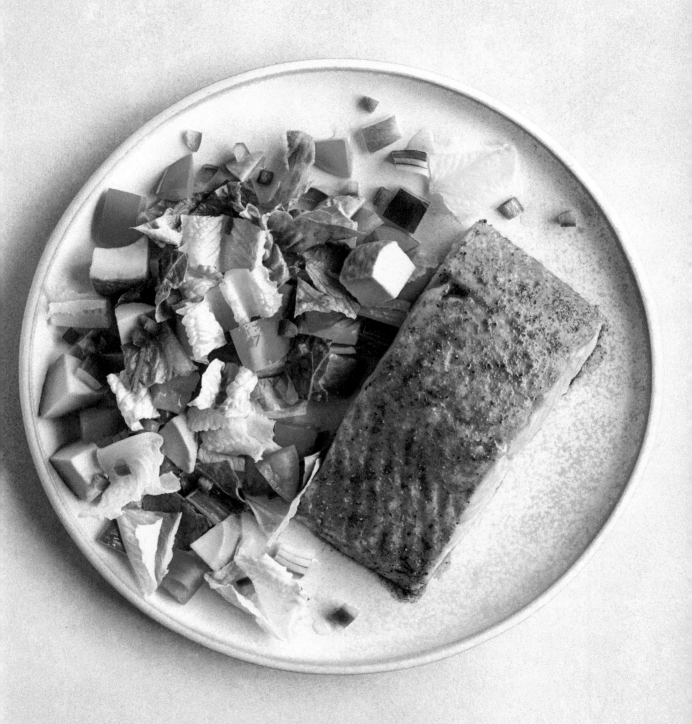

Halibut with Basil Coconut Cream

Egg-Free, Nut-Free
Serves 4 / Prep time: 10 minutes **/ Cook time:** 15 minutes

With a mild and sweet flavor, halibut is a great option for those who don't love the taste of fish. The basil coconut cream sauce enhances the halibut for a tropical-inspired entrée that is perfectly complemented by Mango Salsa (page 136).

FOR THE HALIBUT

4 teaspoons lemon pepper seasoning

1 teaspoon garlic powder

4 (4- to 6-ounce) halibut fillets

3 tablespoons coconut oil or ghee

FOR THE COCONUT CREAM

1 cup full-fat coconut milk

¼ cup freshly squeezed lemon juice (from 2 lemons)

2 teaspoons garlic powder

¼ cup shredded fresh basil leaves

¼ teaspoon sea salt

1. **Make the halibut:** In a small bowl, combine the lemon pepper and garlic powder. Rub the seasoning over both sides of the fish.

2. In a large pan, heat the oil over medium-high heat. Add the halibut and cook until a golden crust forms on the bottom, 3 to 5 minutes. Reduce the heat to medium, flip the fish, and cook until it flakes easily with a fork, about 5 minutes more.

3. **Make the coconut cream:** While the halibut cooks, in a small saucepan, combine the coconut milk, lemon juice, garlic powder, basil, and salt. Bring to a simmer over medium heat, then cook for 2 minutes.

4. Top the halibut with the basil coconut cream and serve.

Ingredient Tip: To make your own AIP-friendly lemon pepper seasoning, combine 1 tablespoon lemon zest with 2 teaspoons freshly ground black pepper and 1 tablespoon sea salt. Freeze any leftover seasoning for later use.

....

Per Serving (about 5 ounces halibut with ¼ cup coconut cream):
Calories: 332; Total Fat: 24g; Protein: 28g; Carbohydrates: 3g; Fiber: 0g

Turmeric Trout with Roasted Carrots

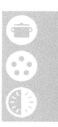

Egg-Free, Nut-Free
Serves 2 / Prep time: 5 minutes / **Cook time:** 25 minutes

Popular for its antioxidant and anti-inflammatory benefits, turmeric is nature's medicine. For maximum absorption, consume turmeric with fat and a pinch of black pepper, as we do in this recipe.

FOR THE ROASTED CARROTS

1 pound carrots
1 tablespoon avocado oil
½ teaspoon sea salt

FOR THE TROUT

1½ tablespoons melted ghee or avocado oil
½ teaspoon ground turmeric
½ teaspoon ground ginger
½ teaspoon sea salt
¼ teaspoon freshly ground black pepper
2 (4- to 6-ounce) trout fillets

1. Preheat the oven to 425°F.

2. **Make the roasted carrots:** Cut the carrots into ½-inch-thick coins (you should have about 3 cups). Place them on a rimmed baking sheet. Coat the carrots with the oil and season with the salt. Roast for 15 minutes, then remove from the oven. Set aside.

3. **Make the trout:** While the carrots are roasting, in a small bowl, mix the ghee, turmeric, ginger, salt, and pepper. Rub the mixture onto all sides of the trout.

4. Add the trout to the pan with the roasted carrots, skin-side down. Return the baking sheet to the oven and roast for about 10 minutes, until the trout flakes easily with a fork.

5. Enjoy the trout with the roasted carrots on the side.

Smart Shopping: Buy frequently used spices in bulk to save money and ensure freshness.

Per Serving (1 trout fillet and 1½ cups carrots): Calories: 383; Total Fat: 22g; Protein: 24g; Carbohydrates: 22g; Fiber: 6g

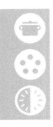

Coconut-Poached Sea Bass

AIP, Egg-Free, Nut-Free
Serves 4 / Prep time: 5 minutes / **Cook time:** 15 minutes

You won't believe the buttery flavor you can create by poaching fish in coconut oil. Sea bass has a mild taste and meaty texture, similar to halibut. Also, like halibut, sea bass is a great choice for those who don't love a "fishy" flavor. We enjoy the simplicity of this recipe and believe in keeping it that way by serving it alongside Simple Cauliflower Rice (page 70).

4 (4- to 6-ounce) sea bass fillets
1 teaspoon sea salt
½ cup coconut oil, or enough for ¼-inch depth in your pan

1. Season the sea bass with salt and set aside.

2. In a medium skillet, melt enough coconut oil over medium-low heat to reach a depth of ¼ inch. When the oil starts to shimmer, reduce the heat to very low and add the sea bass. Cover and cook until the bottom half of the fish is opaque, 8 to 10 minutes, then flip and cook for 4 minutes more, or until fish is cooked through and flakes easily with a fork. Enjoy!

Switch It Up: Sea bass can be expensive, especially when it's out of season. You can use any firm white-fleshed fish for this recipe, such as cod, trout, rockfish, or halibut.

Per Serving (about 5 ounces sea bass): Calories: 196; Total Fat: 10g; Protein: 26g; Carbohydrates: 0g; Fiber: 0g

Smoked Salmon Lettuce Rolls

No-Cook, Egg-Free, Nut-Free
Serves 2 / Prep time: 10 minutes

These quick-and-easy rolls are a vibrant addition to any party platter and are bursting with unique flavors, vitamins, and minerals. Tahini is a seed butter made from sesame seeds and is commonly used in Middle Eastern and Mediterranean cooking. Combined with salty coconut aminos and spicy sriracha, this winning combination will delight even the pickiest of palates.

¼ cup tahini

Juice of 1 lemon

1 teaspoon coconut aminos

1½ teaspoons sriracha

8 butter lettuce leaves

1 large avocado

Pinch sea salt

Pinch freshly ground black pepper

6 ounces smoked salmon or lox

1. In a small bowl, combine the tahini, 1 tablespoon of the lemon juice, the coconut aminos, and the sriracha. Mix well to combine.

2. Wash and dry the lettuce leaves and place 4 on each serving plate, stacking 2 leaves for each roll. Slice the avocado and sprinkle with salt and pepper.

3. Divide the sauce, avocado, and salmon evenly among the lettuce leaves. Finish with additional lemon juice and serve.

Switch It Up: Any hot sauce can replace the sriracha in this recipe. Cashew butter or sunflower seed butter can be used in place of the tahini as well.

Per Serving (2 rolls): Calories: 452; Total Fat: 34g; Protein: 24g; Carbohydrates: 18g; Fiber: 10g

Sushi Bites

No-Cook, Egg-Free, Nut-Free
Serves 2 / Prep time: 10 minutes

Looking for a tasty treat tonight? Enjoy an open-faced sushi bite! Salmon, avocado, and crunchy veggies delight—your guests will be happy feeling full yet so light. Nori is healthy and wasabi is hot, and you'll enjoy this sushi, fish lover or not. It doesn't get faster or easier to make than this, as a snack or a lunch, you'll be floating in bliss!

1 medium cucumber

5 radishes

½ avocado

4 scallions (optional)

20 roasted seaweed snacks

4 ounces smoked salmon or lox

¼ teaspoon sea salt

¼ teaspoon freshly ground black pepper

Wasabi paste (optional)

1. Using a sharp knife or a mandoline, thinly slice the cucumber and radishes (you will need 20 slices of each). Slice the avocado into 10 thin pieces. Finely chop the scallions (if using).

2. Arrange the seaweed snacks in stacks of 2 to form a strong base for your toppings. Divide the smoked salmon evenly among the 10 seaweed stacks. Layer each stack with 2 cucumber slices, 2 radish slices, and 1 slice of avocado. Sprinkle with the salt and pepper. Top with a pea-size dot of wasabi, if desired, and some scallions. Enjoy!

Smart Shopping: Purchase SeaSnax brand small nori seaweed snacks for a perfectly bite-size, no-cut option. Alternatively, you can cut larger nori sheets into 2 ¼-by-3-inch pieces.

Per Serving (5 bites): Calories: 203; Total Fat: 13g; Protein: 15g; Carbohydrates: 7g; Fiber: 4g

Spicy Shrimp and Grits

Egg-Free, Nut-Free
Serves 4 / Prep time: 10 minutes / **Cook time:** 10 minutes

Traditional grits are made from cornmeal. Because corn is technically a grain (not a vegetable!), corn and all corn-derived products are not Paleo. For this Southern favorite, we've replaced the corn with Paleo-friendly cauliflower to create irresistible grits that perfectly complement the spicy shrimp.

FOR THE GRITS

8 cups riced cauliflower (see tip on page 46)
1½ cups full-fat coconut milk
1 teaspoon sea salt
½ teaspoon freshly ground black pepper
2 tablespoons ghee

FOR THE SHRIMP

1 pound raw large shrimp, peeled and deveined
2 teaspoons freshly squeezed lime juice (from ½ lime)
1½ teaspoons chili powder
¼ teaspoon sea salt
¼ teaspoon cayenne pepper
1 tablespoon avocado oil or bacon fat

1. **Make the grits:** In a medium saucepan, combine the cauliflower rice, coconut milk, salt, and pepper. Bring to a simmer over medium-high heat, then reduce the heat to low and simmer, stirring occasionally, for 10 minutes, or until the cauliflower is tender. Remove from the heat and stir in the ghee. Cover to keep warm and set aside.

2. **Make the shrimp:** While the grits simmer, in a medium bowl, toss the shrimp with the lime juice, chili powder, salt, and cayenne. In a large skillet, heat the oil over medium-high heat. When the oil is hot, add the shrimp and the juices from the bowl. Cook, stirring occasionally, for 3 to 5 minutes, until the shrimp cooks through and turns pink.

3. Spoon the grits into bowls and top with the shrimp. Drizzle any juices from the pan over the shrimp and grits. Enjoy!

Switch It Up: Prawns also work great in this recipe.

....

Per Serving (1 cup grits and 4 ounces shrimp): Calories: 408; Total Fat: 29g; Protein: 28g; Carbohydrates: 13g; Fiber: 4g

Fiesta Fish Tacos

Egg-Free, Nut-Free
Serves 4 / Prep time: 15 minutes / **Cook time:** 10 minutes

These tasty tacos will rival ones you've had in top-notch seafood restaurants. For extra heat, add diced jalapeños to the slaw. To save time, skip the tapioca breading and just bake the marinated fish strips.

FOR THE FISH
1 pound skinless cod
2 tablespoons ghee
2 tablespoons freshly squeeze lime juice (from 1 lime)
3 tablespoons taco seasoning
½ cup tapioca flour

FOR THE SLAW
2 cups thinly sliced cabbage (⅛ head)
½ bell pepper (any color), thinly sliced
½ red onion, thinly sliced
½ cup chopped fresh cilantro
Juice of 1 lime
¼ teaspoon sea salt
¼ teaspoon freshly ground black pepper
1 large avocado, for garnish
12 large romaine lettuce leaves

1. **Make the fish:** Preheat the oven to 400°F and line a baking sheet with parchment paper.

2. Cut the cod into 1-inch-wide strips. Pat dry and set aside.

3. In a medium microwave-safe bowl, melt the ghee in the microwave. In the same bowl, combine the melted ghee, lime juice, and taco seasoning to make the marinade. Put the tapioca flour in another medium bowl. Dip each piece of fish in the marinade, then dredge in the tapioca flour to coat all sides. Place the coated fish strips on the prepared baking sheet. Bake for 10 to 15 minutes, until the breading turns a light golden brown.

4. **Make the slaw:** Combine the cabbage, bell pepper, and onion in a large bowl. Add the cilantro, lime juice, salt, and pepper and combine. Slice the avocado.

5. Fill each lettuce leaf with slaw, fish, and avocado slices. Serve extra slaw on the side.

Switch It Up: If you prefer your tacos on tortillas, try making our Paleo Tortillas (page 160) or purchase Paleo-friendly Siete Foods tortillas, which can be fried in avocado oil into a perfectly crispy taco shell.

....

Per Serving (2 or 3 tacos): Calories: 287; Total Fat: 15g; Protein: 22g; Carbohydrates: 17g; Fiber: 5g

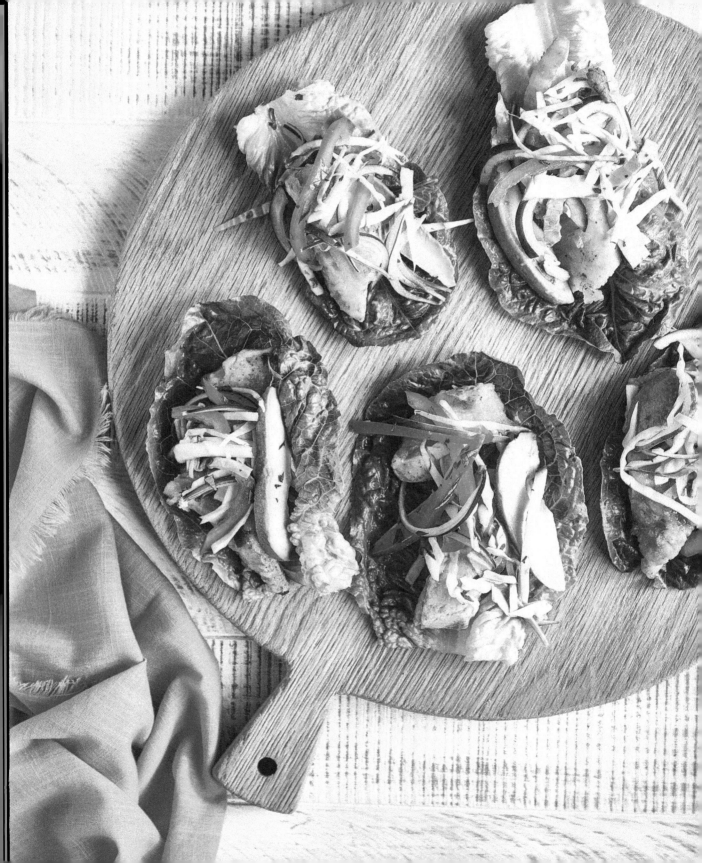

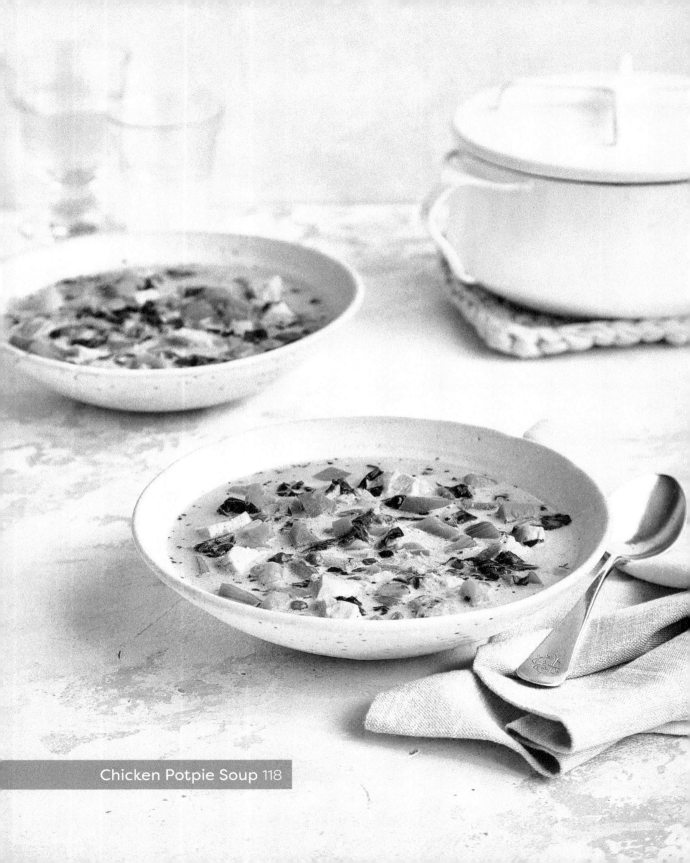

Chicken Potpie Soup 118

CHAPTER 6

Poultry

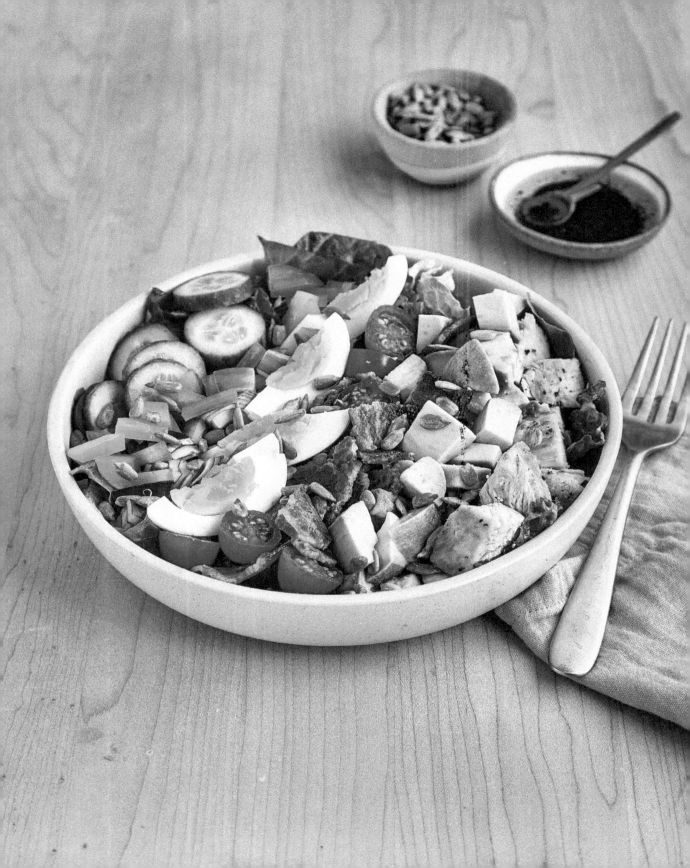

Rainbow Power Bowl

Nut-Free
Serves 4 / Prep time: 15 minutes / **Cook time:** 15 minutes

This Cobb salad spin-off will delight both your palate and your eyes. Each bite of this cool, crisp salad boasts a rainbow of color: red tomato, orange bell pepper, yellow yolks, green cucumber, and purple onion. Most Paleo dieters have cooked bacon and hard-boiled eggs on hand in the refrigerator, and this recipe is a great way to use them up. Steps 1 through 4 of this recipe can be done simultaneously to save time.

1 pound boneless, skinless chicken breasts
Seasoning of choice (such as Italian seasoning, poultry seasoning, salt and pepper)
8 bacon slices
4 large eggs
1 head romaine lettuce
1 orange bell pepper
1 cucumber
1 large avocado
½ red onion
1 cup cherry tomatoes
Extra-virgin olive oil
Balsamic vinegar
¼ cup toasted and hulled sunflower seeds
Pinch sea salt
Pinch freshly ground black pepper

1. Put the chicken breasts and your seasoning of choice in a medium pot and add enough water or broth to cover. Bring to a boil over medium-high heat, then reduce the heat to maintain a simmer, cover, and cook for 8 to 15 minutes, until a thermometer inserted into the thickest part of the meat registers 165°F. Remove the chicken from the poaching liquid and set aside on a cutting board to cool briefly, then slice.

2. Preheat the oven to 400°F. Line a baking sheet with aluminum foil or parchment paper. Arrange the bacon on the prepared baking sheet so the slices aren't touching and bake for 15 to 20 minutes, to your desired crispiness.

3. Place a steamer basket in a medium pot and add enough water to reach the bottom of the basket. Cover and bring to a boil over high heat. Add the eggs, cover, and steam for 13 minutes. Transfer the eggs to an ice bath until cool.

continued →

4. While the bacon, eggs, and chicken are cooking, chop the lettuce into 1-inch strips (you should have about 8 cups). Slice the bell pepper, cucumber, avocado, and onion. Halve the tomatoes.

5. Cut the chicken into ½-inch cubes. Peel and quarter the hard-boiled eggs. Crumble the bacon or cut it into bite-size pieces.

6. Divide all the ingredients among four large salad bowls. Drizzle with oil and vinegar, top with the sunflower seeds, and season with salt and pepper, then serve.

Ingredient Tip: Transform this into a superfast meal by purchasing chopped lettuce, cooked bacon, rotisserie chicken, and hard-boiled eggs. Get creative with your ingredients by adding olives, carrot ribbons, artichoke hearts, jicama, fresh berries, watercress, and more.

Per Serving (3 cups): Calories: 509; Total Fat: 28g; Protein: 45g; Carbohydrates: 20g; Fiber: 9g

Chicken Waldorf Salad

No-Cook
Serves 4 / Prep time: 10 minutes

Waldorf salad was created more than 100 years ago by a maître d' at the Waldorf Astoria hotel in New York City. It was a smash hit at the time, and still is today. The key ingredients are apples, celery, nuts, and mayonnaise, so not much needs to change to make this salad perfectly Paleo.

3 cups diced cooked or rotisserie chicken breast or thighs

1 large apple, cored and chopped into ½-inch pieces

½ cup seedless red or green grapes, halved

1 medium celery stalk, thinly sliced

2 tablespoons chopped fresh basil or parsley

⅓ cup Paleo mayonnaise

½ cup walnut halves

2 tablespoons freshly squeezed lemon juice (from 1 lemon)

Pinch sea salt

Pinch freshly ground black pepper

1 head butter lettuce, leaves separated

1. In a large bowl, mix the chicken, apple, grapes, celery, basil, mayonnaise, walnuts, and lemon juice until combined. Season with the salt and pepper.

2. Divide the chicken salad evenly among the lettuce leaves and enjoy.

Switch It Up: Make your Waldorf salad vegetarian by leaving out the chicken.

Per Serving (1¾ cups salad): Calories: 443; Total Fat: 24g; Protein: 36g; Carbohydrates: 18g; Fiber: 4g

Chicken No-Tortilla Soup

Egg-Free, Nut-Free
Serves 4 / Prep time: 5 minutes / **Cook time:** 30 minutes

Enjoy the high-quality protein, antioxidant-rich veggies, herbs, and spices of tortilla soup, without the unhealthy corn tortilla strips. For some added crunch, top with jicama strips or toasted pumpkin seeds, or serve with a few Paleo-friendly grain-free chips on the side.

4 cups chicken broth

1 pound boneless, skinless chicken breasts or thighs

1 (14-ounce) can diced fire-roasted tomatoes, with their juices

1 (4-ounce) can green chiles, drained

1 teaspoon ground cumin

1 teaspoon garlic powder

½ teaspoon sea salt

2 large carrots

1 large bell pepper

2 cups baby spinach or shredded cabbage

1 tablespoon freshly squeezed lime juice (from ½ lime)

½ cup fresh cilantro, for garnish

2 jalapeños, for garnish

1 avocado, for garnish

1. In a large pot, combine the broth, chicken, tomatoes and their juices, chiles, cumin, garlic powder, and salt. Bring to a boil over medium-high heat, then reduce the heat to low, cover, and simmer for 20 minutes, until the chicken is cooked through.

2. While the chicken cooks, chop the carrots, bell pepper, and cilantro. Slice the jalapeños and avocado. Set aside.

3. Transfer the chicken to a cutting board. Using two forks, shred the meat, then return it to the pot. Add the carrots, bell pepper, spinach, and lime juice and simmer, uncovered, for 10 minutes, or until the veggies are soft.

4. Ladle into bowls, garnish with the cilantro, jalapeños, and avocado, and enjoy!

Switch It Up: Soups are fantastic opportunities to incorporate bone broth into your diet. Switch out the chicken broth for Homemade Bone Broth (page 168) or your favorite store-bought brand.

....

Per Serving (2 cups): Calories: 314; Total Fat: 8g; Protein: 31g; Carbohydrates: 21g; Fiber: 8g

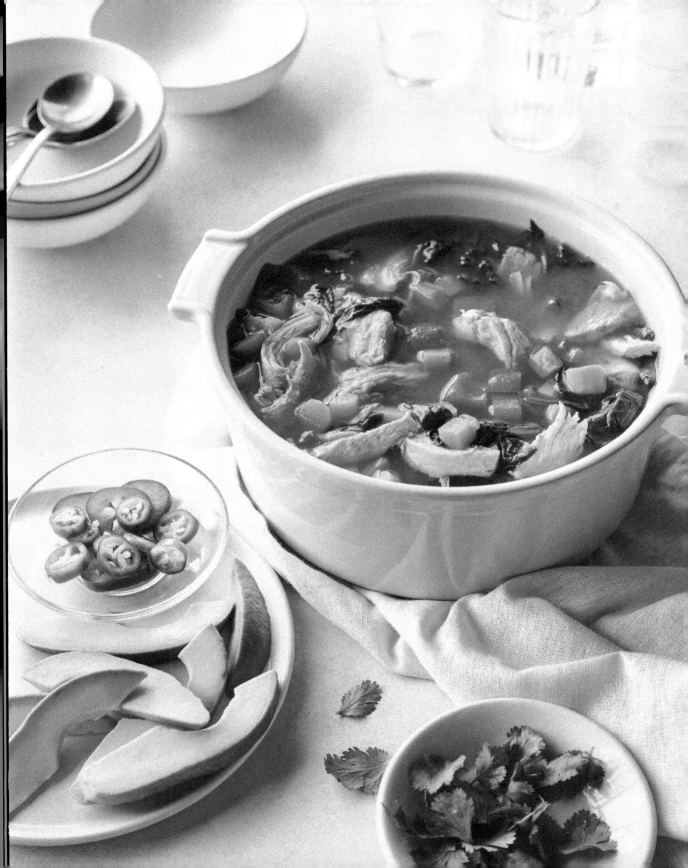

Kickin' Chicken Strips

Serves 4 / Prep time: 10 minutes **/ Cook time:** 20 minutes

No one will miss the drive-through when you serve up these flavorful grain-free chicken strips. Serve them with Sweet Potato Fries (page 64) and a side of Tomato Ketchup (page 164) for dipping.

⅓ cup tapioca flour or arrowroot flour

3 large egg whites, beaten

1 cup almond flour

1¼ teaspoons paprika

1¼ teaspoons ground cumin

1 teaspoon garlic powder

1 teaspoon sea salt

1 teaspoon freshly ground black pepper

¼ teaspoon cayenne pepper (optional)

1½ pounds boneless, skinless chicken breasts

1. Preheat the oven to 375°F. Line a large baking sheet with parchment paper.

2. Arrange three shallow bowls in a row on the counter. Put the tapioca flour in the first and the egg whites in the second; in the third bowl, mix the almond flour, paprika, cumin, garlic powder, salt, pepper, and cayenne (if using).

3. Pat the chicken dry with a paper towel, then slice it crosswise into 1-inch-wide strips.

4. In assembly line fashion, dredge a chicken strip through the tapioca flour to coat, then dip it into the egg whites, and finally dredge it through the almond flour mixture. Place the breaded chicken strip on the prepared baking sheet. Repeat to bread the remaining chicken.

5. Bake for 20 to 25 minutes, until the chicken strips are lightly browned. Serve warm.

Serving Tip: If you won't be serving the chicken strips immediately, transfer them to a wire rack to cool. This prevents them from becoming soggy on the bottom.

Per Serving (4 ounces): Calories: 302; Total Fat: 12g; Protein: 42g; Carbohydrates: 7g; Fiber: 2g

Butternut Bacon-Wrapped Chicken Thighs

AIP, Egg-Free, Nut-Free
Serves 4 / Prep time: 15 minutes / **Cook time:** 40 minutes

We use a 9-by-13-inch casserole dish for this winning one-pan recipe to allow bacon to infuse its flavor. Save time by purchasing peeled and cubed butternut squash.

1 (2½- to 3-pound) butternut squash

1 tablespoon avocado oil

8 skinless chicken thighs (bone-in or boneless)

1 teaspoon sea salt

½ teaspoon freshly ground black pepper

8 bacon slices, plus more if needed

1. Preheat the oven to 375°F.

2. With a vegetable peeler, remove the skin from the squash. Using a large chef's knife, halve the squash, remove the seeds, and cut the flesh into 1-inch cubes (you should have about 5 cups). Transfer the squash to a 9-by-13-inch casserole dish. Add the avocado oil and toss to coat.

3. Season the chicken with the salt and pepper. Wrap each piece with a slice of bacon (you can use a second slice of bacon to wrap larger chicken thighs, if needed). Place the bacon-wrapped chicken on top of the butternut squash in the casserole dish.

4. Bake for 40 minutes, or until the internal temperature of the chicken reaches 165°F, and the squash is tender. Serve hot and enjoy!

Technique Tip: Remove skin from skin-on chicken thighs for this recipe. Fry it up for a delicious, collagen-packed snack!

Per Serving (2 pieces chicken and about 1¼ cups butternut squash): Calories: 492; Total Fat: 21g; Protein: 54g; Carbohydrates: 21g; Fiber: 4g

Turkey Wraps

No-Cook, Nut-Free
Serves 2 / Prep time: 10 minutes

No need to miss sandwiches! Paleo lunch doesn't get much better (or easier) than lettuce wraps. These are extra special, thanks to the tangy addition of dill pickles. If you're not a fan of pickles, any fermented condiment, such as sauerkraut or kimchi, will work. Bonus: Your gut will love the probiotics!

4 small tomatoes, such as Roma (plum)

¼ cup fresh basil leaves

2 tablespoons Paleo mayonnaise, divided

4 large romaine lettuce, cabbage, or stemmed chard leaves

8 ounces sliced deli turkey

⅓ cup dill pickle slices

1. Thinly slice the tomatoes. Shred the basil. Set aside.

2. Spread 1½ teaspoons of the mayonnaise on each lettuce leaf. Layer with the turkey, tomato, and basil, dividing them evenly among the lettuce leaves. Top with the pickle slices.

3. Fold the leaves in half lengthwise and enjoy!

Smart Shopping: Choose the highest-quality lunch meat your budget allows. This means looking for brands that contain no unwanted additives and preservatives while supporting the sustainable and ethical treatment of animals. One of our favorite brands is Applegate.

Per Serving (2 wraps): Calories: 311; Total Fat: 17g; Protein: 25g; Carbohydrates: 16g; Fiber: 6g

Turkey Burgers on Portobello Buns

Nut-Free
Serves 4 / Prep time: 10 minutes / **Cook time:** 20 minutes

Portobellos make great grain-free buns, while providing plenty of nutrients and antioxidants. You can serve these on large lettuce leaves instead.

FOR THE CHIPOTLE MAYO

½ cup Paleo mayonnaise

¾ teaspoon ground chipotle chile

Juice of 1 lime

FOR THE TURKEY BURGERS

4 portobello mushroom caps

1½ pounds ground turkey

1 teaspoon garlic powder

½ teaspoon onion powder

½ teaspoon ground cumin

¼ teaspoon red pepper flakes

1 teaspoon sea salt

1 tablespoon avocado oil

2 large tomatoes, sliced

2 cups arugula

1. Preheat the oven to 425°F. Line a baking sheet with parchment paper.

2. **Make the chipotle mayo:** In a small bowl, stir together the mayonnaise, chipotle, and lime juice. Set aside.

3. **Make the turkey burgers:** Put the mushroom caps on the prepared baking sheet, gill-side down. Bake for 15 minutes, or until softened. Transfer to a paper towel–lined plate.

4. In a medium bowl, mix the turkey, garlic powder, onion powder, cumin, red pepper flakes, and salt. Form the turkey mixture into four patties.

5. In a large pan, heat the oil over medium heat. Add the turkey burgers. Cook until the burgers are browned and cooked through, about 10 minutes per side.

6. Place a burger on each mushroom cap and top each with 1 to 2 tablespoons of the chipotle mayo, one-quarter of the tomato slices, and ½ cup of the arugula.

Per Serving (1 burger): Calories: 480; Total Fat: 35g; Protein: 36g; Carbohydrates: 9g; Fiber: 2g

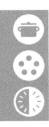

One-Pan Chicken and Chard

AIP, Egg-Free, Nut-Free
Serves 4 / Prep time: 5 minutes **/ Cook time:** 20 minutes

If you have a cast-iron skillet, use it for this recipe and enjoy the benefit of extra iron in your meal. A well-seasoned cast-iron pan is also a great option for recipes that start on the stovetop and finish in the oven.

2 tablespoons
   avocado oil
4 bone-in, skin-on
   chicken thighs
1 large sweet potato,
   cut into ½-inch cubes
1½ teaspoons sea salt,
   divided
1 teaspoon freshly
   ground black pepper
2 garlic cloves, minced
4 cups chopped
   stemmed chard
   leaves

1. Preheat the oven to 425°F.

2. In a large oven-safe pan, heat the oil over medium heat. Place the chicken in the pan, skin-side down, and arrange the sweet potatoes around the chicken. Season the contents of the pan with 1 teaspoon of salt and the pepper. Cook, stirring only the potatoes occasionally, until the chicken skin is golden brown and crisp, 10 to 15 minutes.

3. Flip the thighs and transfer the pan to the oven. Bake for 8 to 10 minutes, until the chicken is cooked through, and the sweet potatoes are soft. Transfer the pan back to the stovetop. Transfer the chicken and sweet potatoes to serving plates, leaving the drippings in the pan.

4. Add the garlic to the pan and cook over low heat, stirring, for 1 minute. Add the chard and remaining ½ teaspoon salt. Cook, stirring continuously, until wilted, about 2 minutes.

5. Enjoy the chard alongside the chicken and sweet potatoes.

Appliance Tip: A cast-iron skillet, oven-safe stainless-steel pan, or Dutch oven will work for this recipe.

....

Per Serving (1 chicken thigh, 1 cup sweet potatoes, and ½ cup chard): Calories: 299; Total Fat: 21g; Protein: 19g; Carbohydrates: 11g; Fiber: 2g

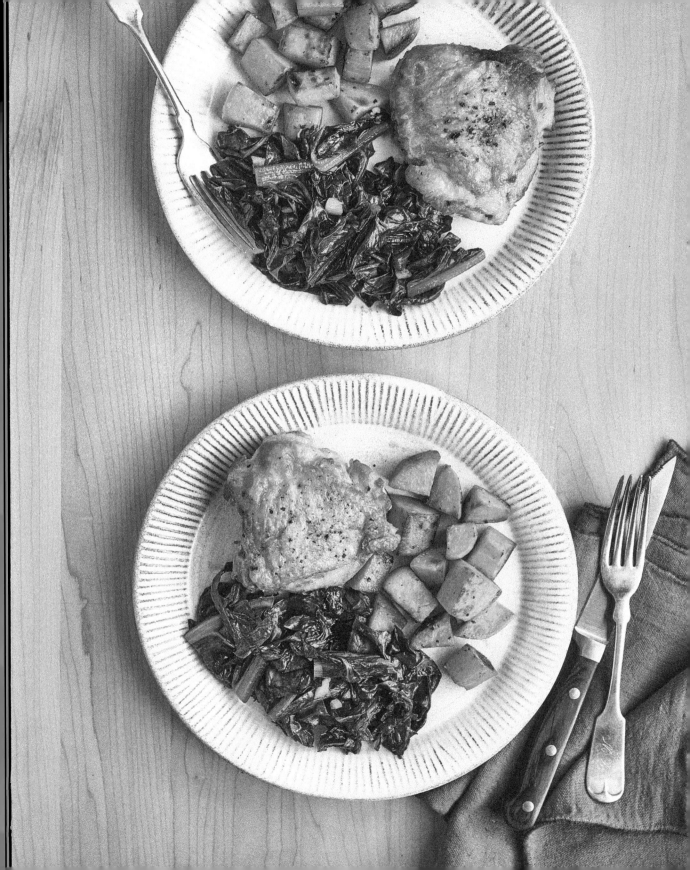

Chicken Veggie Stir-Fry

Egg-Free, Nut-Free
Serves 4 / Prep time: 15 minutes / **Cook time:** 10 minutes

We love using coconut aminos in stir-fries. They taste just like soy sauce but are made from coconut blossoms, so they're perfectly Paleo.

2 garlic cloves

2 scallions

1 pound baby bok choy

4 cups broccoli florets

1 tablespoon
avocado oil

1 teaspoon minced or
grated fresh ginger

4 ounces green beans

1 cup sliced mushrooms

2 tablespoons coconut
aminos

1 tablespoon freshly
squeezed lime juice
(from ½ lime)

1 tablespoon fish sauce
(optional)

3 cups sliced or cubed
cooked or rotisserie
chicken

1 tablespoon toasted
sesame oil

1. Mince the garlic and chop the scallions. Chop the bok choy into 1-inch pieces. Cut the broccoli florets into bite-size pieces.

2. In a large skillet or wok, heat the avocado oil over medium heat. When hot, add the garlic, scallions, and ginger. Cook for 1 to 2 minutes, stirring frequently, until fragrant. Add the bok choy, broccoli, green beans, mushrooms, coconut aminos, lime juice, and fish sauce (if using). Cook, stirring frequently, for 6 to 8 minutes, until the vegetables are crisp-tender. Stir in the chicken and sesame oil and cook for 3 to 5 minutes more, until the chicken is warmed through. Enjoy hot.

Switch It Up: Try swapping in leftover pork or beef for the chicken to change things up. If you can't find baby bok choy in your market, a pound of carrots or bell peppers (sliced) substitute beautifully.

Per Serving: Calories: 270; Total Fat: 11g; Protein: 32g; Carbohydrates: 10g; Fiber: 3g

Sheet Pan Fajitas with Coconut-Lime Dressing

Egg-Free, Nut-Free
Serves 4 / Prep time: 10 minutes / **Cook time:** 20 minutes

One-pan recipes come together quickly and clean up just as fast. Serve on leafy greens such as chard, cabbage, collards, or lettuce, or on Paleo Tortillas (page 160). The coconut-lime dressing adds a bright and citrusy finish to this kickin' dish.

FOR THE SPICE BLEND
2 teaspoons chili powder
2 teaspoons ground cumin
2 teaspoons garlic powder
2 teaspoons onion powder
½ teaspoon sea salt
½ teaspoon freshly ground black pepper

FOR THE FAJITAS
1 pound boneless, skinless turkey breast
2 large bell peppers
1 medium yellow onion
2 tablespoons avocado oil →

1. Preheat the oven to 400°F. Line a baking sheet with parchment paper.

2. **Make the spice blend:** In a small bowl, mix the chili powder, cumin, garlic powder, onion powder, salt, and pepper.

3. **Make the fajitas:** Cut the turkey, bell peppers, and onion into ½-inch-thick slices. Combine them in a large bowl with the oil and spice blend and toss to coat.

4. Pour the turkey and veggies onto the baking sheet. Bake for 20 minutes, or until the turkey is cooked through and the veggies are soft.

continued →

FOR THE COCONUT-LIME DRESSING

½ cup full-fat coconut milk

Juice of 1 lime

1 teaspoon apple cider vinegar

¼ teaspoon garlic powder

TO SERVE

1 head romaine lettuce, leaves separated

¼ cup chopped fresh cilantro, for garnish

5. **Make the coconut-lime dressing:** In a small bowl, stir together the coconut milk, lime juice, vinegar, and garlic powder.

6. Serve the turkey and veggies in the lettuce leaves, drizzled with dressing, garnished with the cilantro. Store leftover dressing in an airtight container in the refrigerator for up to 1 week.

Smart Shopping: Purchase premade fajita seasoning to save time. We love Riega Foods organic chicken fajita seasoning.

....

Per Serving (1½ cups fajitas and 2 tablespoons dressing): Calories: 342; Total Fat: 16g; Protein: 31g; Carbohydrates: 17g; Fiber: 6g

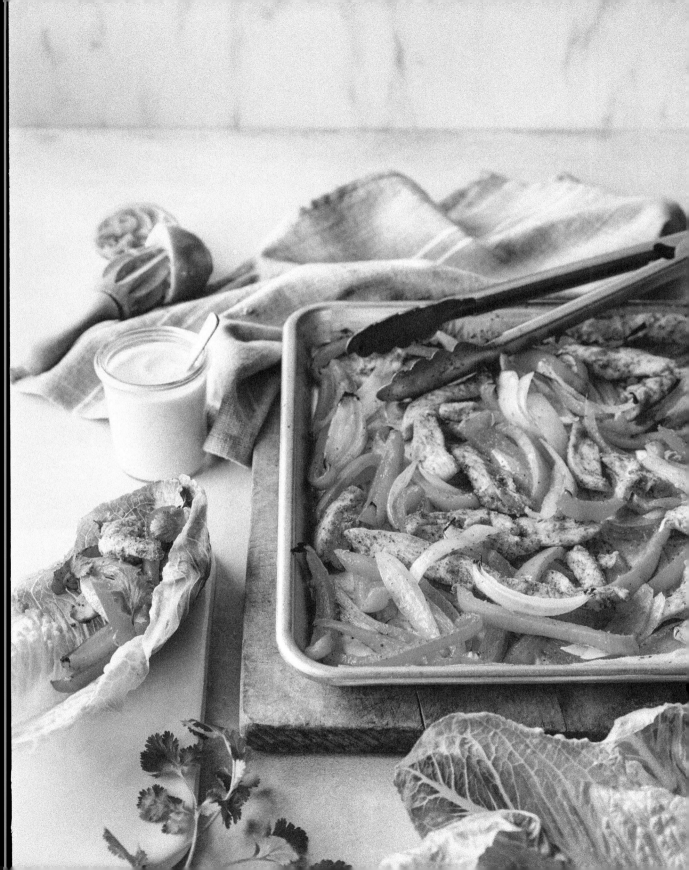

Chicken Potpie Soup

Egg-Free, Nut-Free
Serves 6 / Prep time: 5 minutes / **Cook time:** 30 minutes

This easy, creamy potpie soup is the ultimate comfort food. A classic potpie ingredient is green peas, which are classified as legumes (beans). They are, however, allowed on the Paleo diet because they are lower in gut-irritating antinutrients (e.g., phytates and lectins) compared to most other legumes. Green beans, snap peas, and snow peas are all considered Paleo-friendly in moderation. If you prefer, swap out the peas for broccoli florets instead.

2 tablespoons
    avocado oil
1 onion, chopped
2 garlic cloves, minced
3 cups chicken broth
1 pound boneless,
    skinless chicken
    breasts or thighs
1 tablespoon Italian
    seasoning
1 teaspoon dried thyme
1 teaspoon sea salt
½ teaspoon freshly
    ground black pepper
1 (13.5-ounce) can
    full-fat coconut milk
2 carrots, chopped
1 sweet potato,
    chopped
1 celery stalk, chopped
4 cups baby spinach or
    chopped fresh parsley
1 cup frozen green peas

1. In a large pot, heat the oil over medium heat. Add the onion and garlic and cook, stirring, until lightly browned, 1 to 2 minutes. Add the broth, chicken, Italian seasoning, thyme, salt, and pepper. Bring to a boil, then reduce the heat to low, cover, and simmer for 20 minutes.

2. Transfer the chicken to a cutting board and carefully chop it into cubes, then return it to the pot. Stir in the coconut milk, carrots, sweet potato, celery, spinach, and peas. Cover and simmer for about 10 minutes, until the veggies are soft.

Technique Tip: To thicken this soup, whisk in 1 to 2 tablespoons tapioca flour or arrowroot flour along with the coconut milk in step 2.

Per Serving (1½ cups): Calories: 320; Total Fat: 21g; Protein: 21g; Carbohydrates: 14g; Fiber: 3g

Meat Lovers' Ratatouille

Egg-Free, Nut-Free
Serves 4 / Prep time: 10 minutes **/ Cook time:** 40 minutes

Ratatouille is a traditional French stew that turns an ordinary array of vegetables into a culinary treat. Classic ratatouille features eggplant, bell pepper, and tomato, which are nightshade vegetables. If you are sensitive to nightshades, replace them with any veggies you like. Omit the meat to make this vegan.

1 pound boneless, skinless chicken breast
1 pound Italian sausage
1 tablespoon extra-virgin olive oil
1 teaspoon sea salt
1 medium eggplant
1 bell pepper
1 medium zucchini
1 medium summer squash
1 medium yellow onion
2 large tomatoes
1 tablespoon Italian seasoning
2 tablespoons thinly sliced fresh basil leaves, for garnish

1. Slice the chicken into bite-size pieces. If your sausage is in links, remove the casings.

2. In a large pot, heat the oil over medium heat. Add the chicken, sausage, and salt and cook, stirring occasionally and leaving the sausage in bite-size chunks, for 10 minutes, or until they start to brown.

3. While the meat is cooking, chop the eggplant, bell pepper, zucchini, squash, onion, and tomatoes into large dice.

4. Add the vegetables and Italian seasoning to the pot with the meat and stir to combine. Reduce the heat to low, cover, and cook, stirring occasionally, for 30 to 35 minutes, until the vegetables are tender.

5. Garnish with the basil and enjoy.

Love Your Leftovers: Reheat leftovers in a pan with shredded sweet potato and ghee to make yourself a spectacular breakfast hash. Top with a fried egg for a meal that will carry you through the day!

Per Serving (2 cups): Calories: 378; Total Fat: 17g; Protein: 36g; Carbohydrates: 20g; Fiber: 3g

BBQ Smoky Wings

Egg-Free, Nut-Free
Serves 4 / Prep time: 5 minutes / **Cook time:** 30 minutes

Most barbecue sauces contain unhealthy amounts of sugar and other artificial ingredients. Here the natural sweetness of tomato paste is all you need to create a delicious and healthy barbecue sauce that's perfectly balanced by smoky chipotle and paprika. Serve these wings with carrot and celery sticks and Sweet Potato Fries (page 64).

FOR THE WINGS

24 chicken wings or drumettes

1 teaspoon sea salt

½ teaspoon freshly ground black pepper

FOR THE BARBECUE SAUCE

1 (6-ounce) can tomato paste

½ cup water

¼ cup apple cider vinegar

2 tablespoons Dijon mustard

1 teaspoon garlic powder

1 teaspoon onion powder

½ teaspoon paprika

¼ teaspoon ground chipotle chile

1 teaspoon coconut aminos

1. Preheat the oven to 425°F. Set a wire rack over a rimmed baking sheet.

2. **Make the wings:** Arrange the wings on the rack and pat dry with a paper towel. Season with the salt and pepper. Roast for about 30 minutes, until the internal temperature reaches 165°F, the wings are golden, and their skin is crispy.

3. **Make the barbecue sauce:** In a small saucepan, combine the tomato paste, water, vinegar, mustard, garlic powder, onion powder, paprika, chipotle, and coconut aminos. Cook over low-medium heat, stirring occasionally, until warmed through. Cover and keep warm over very low heat until the wings are done.

4. Remove the wings from the oven and brush with the sauce. Serve the wings with the remaining sauce on the side.

Smart Shopping: To save time, purchase a prepared Paleo-friendly barbecue sauce. One of our favorites is Primal Kitchen Classic BBQ Sauce.

....

Per Serving (6 wings and ¼ cup sauce): Calories: 390; Total Fat: 24g; Protein: 29g; Carbohydrates: 10g; Fiber: 3g

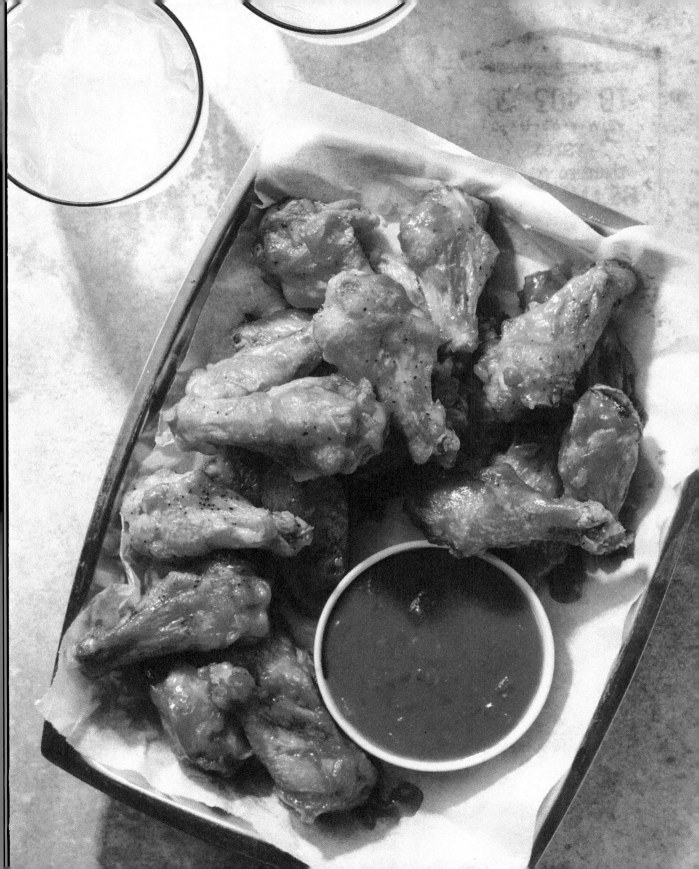

Savory Slow-Cooker Drumsticks

Egg-Free, Nut-Free
Serves 6 / Prep time: 5 minutes / **Cook time:** 3 hours

It's easy to make fantastic chicken drumsticks in your slow cooker, and you don't even need any liquid in the pot! To save time on this recipe, refrigerate prepped chicken in the slow cooker insert the night before (or up to 3 days in advance). When you are ready, just pop it in the cooker and you're free to go run errands while your drumsticks cook. When you return home, your house will smell divine, and dinner will be ready!

1 tablespoon paprika
2 teaspoons garlic powder
2 teaspoons sea salt
1 teaspoon freshly ground black pepper
3 pounds chicken drumsticks

1. In a small bowl, mix the paprika, garlic powder, salt, and pepper.

2. Rub the spice mixture all over each drumstick and place in the slow cooker. Cover and cook on High for 3 to 4 hours or on Low for 6 to 7 hours, until a thermometer inserted into the meaty portion of a drumstick reaches 165°F.

3. Enjoy hot or at room temperature with your favorite Paleo sides.

Switch It Up: Try using different spice blends for variety. Instead of paprika and garlic powder, try cinnamon and chili powder, or sage and onion powder. There are endless combinations of spices to enjoy. Have fun getting creative!

....

Per Serving (2 drumsticks): Calories: 415; Total Fat: 23g; Protein: 50g; Carbohydrates: 1g; Fiber: 0g

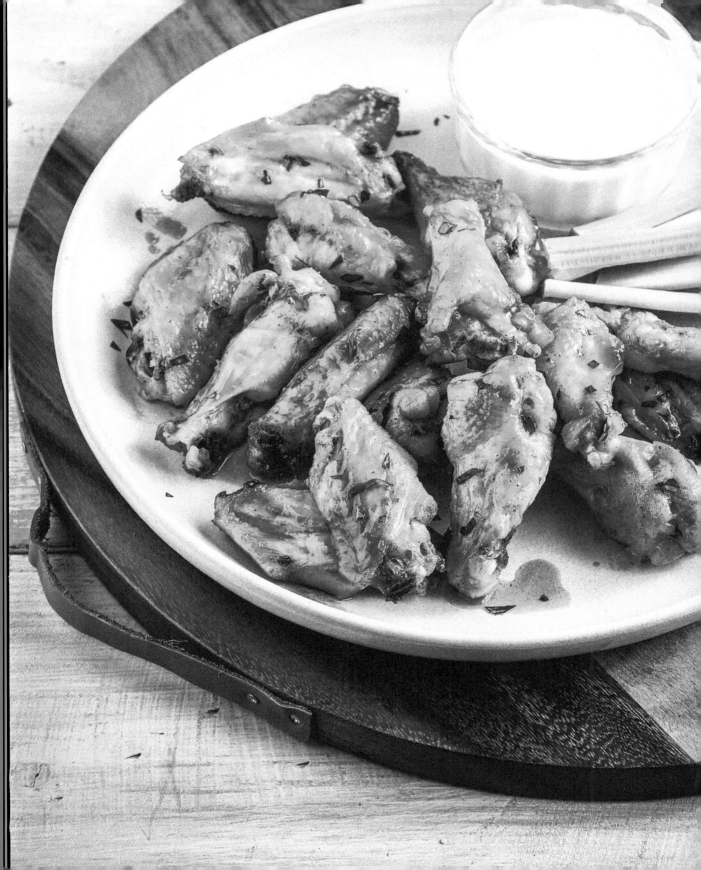

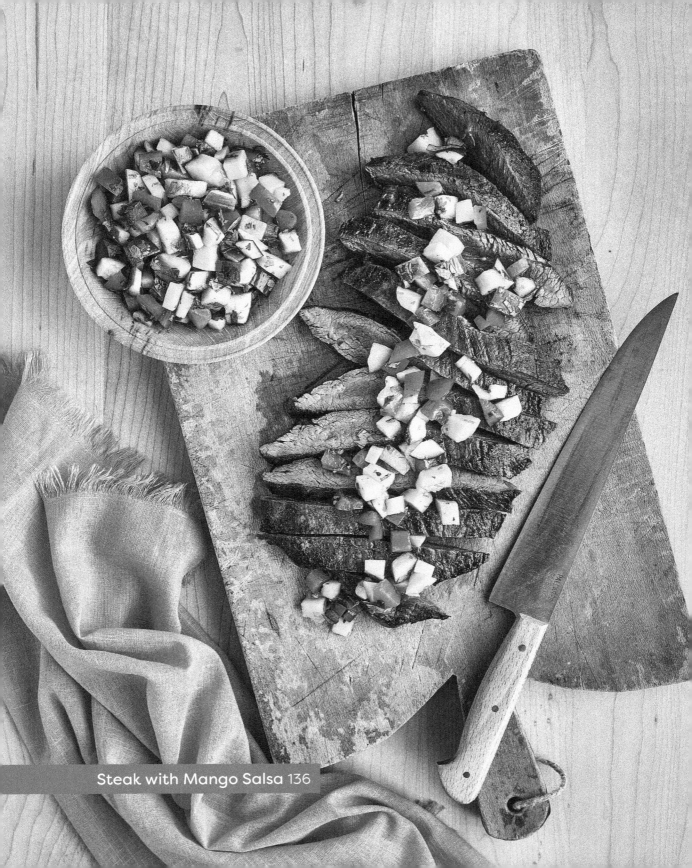

Steak with Mango Salsa 136

CHAPTER 7

Beef, Pork, and Lamb

Ham and Baby Kale Salad

No-Cook, Egg-Free, Nut-Free
Serves 2 / Prep time: 10 minutes

Kale comes in many shapes and sizes, but the most common types are curly kale, Tuscan kale (also known as dinosaur or lacinato kale), and baby kale. All varieties have sturdy leaves and top-notch nutritional profiles. Kale is rich in beta-carotene, vitamin C, vitamin K, folate, calcium, magnesium, and more. Its spicy, bitter flavor is offset beautifully in this salad by the salty ham, soothing avocado, and tart vinegar.

FOR THE DRESSING
2 tablespoons extra-virgin olive oil
2 tablespoons apple cider vinegar
Pinch sea salt
Pinch freshly ground black pepper

FOR THE SALAD
8 ounces cooked ham
2 medium tomatoes
1 medium avocado
6 cups baby kale

1. **Make the dressing:** In a small bowl, mix the oil, vinegar, salt, and pepper. Set aside.

2. **Make the salad:** Chop the ham, tomatoes, and avocado into bite-size pieces. In a large bowl, combine the ham, tomatoes, avocado, and kale. Add the dressing and toss to coat completely. Enjoy!

Switch It Up: Use any variety of kale that you find at your market, or substitute another leafy green, such as chard or spinach; just trim off the tough stems and chop the leaves if it's not a baby variety. If you're in the mood for a really spicy leafy green, try mustard greens, but don't say we didn't warn you!

Per Serving (3½ cups): Calories: 514; Total Fat: 38g; Protein: 23g; Carbohydrates: 22g; Fiber: 11g

Beef-tastic Tacos

Egg-Free, Nut-Free
Serves 4 / Prep time: 5 minutes / **Cook time:** 15 minutes

This taco meat is superflavorful and provides a bit of a kick, but the tomatoes and avocados cool down your palate. If you don't love spice, you can eliminate or reduce the amount of cayenne, remove the seeds and white interior veins of the jalapeño, or both. Make this taco filling to your taste.

1½ pounds ground beef
2 teaspoons chili powder
2 teaspoons ground cumin
2 teaspoons garlic powder
2 teaspoons onion powder
1 teaspoon sea salt
½ teaspoon freshly ground black pepper
½ teaspoon cayenne pepper (optional)
½ cup water
2 large tomatoes
1 medium avocado
1 large jalapeño (optional)
8 large leaves of romaine lettuce, stemmed chard or kale, or cabbage

1. In a large pan, cook the ground beef over medium-high heat, stirring occasionally, for about 8 minutes, until almost browned.

2. While the meat cooks, in a small bowl, mix the chili powder, cumin, garlic powder, onion powder, salt, pepper, and cayenne (if using). When the meat is almost browned, pour the spice mixture into the pan, add the water, and stir to combine. Simmer, uncovered, for about 5 minutes, until the meat is cooked through.

3. While the meat and spices simmer, chop the tomatoes, avocado, and jalapeño (if using).

4. Divide the taco meat among the lettuce leaves and top with the tomatoes, avocado, and jalapeño, if using.

Smart Shopping: To save time on this recipe, use a premade taco seasoning. We love taco seasoning from Trader Joe's and Riega Foods.

....

Per Serving (2 tacos): Calories: 339; Total Fat: 17g; Protein: 39g; Carbohydrates: 11g; Fiber: 6g

So-Good Sloppy Joes

Egg-Free, Nut-Free
Serves 4 / Prep time: 5 minutes / **Cook time:** 15 minutes

According to legend, the sloppy joe was born nearly a century ago when a cook named Joe mixed some tomato sauce into ground beef and served it on a bun. More recently, processed-food manufacturers added sugar to the tomato sauce, creating a sweet sloppy joe. Here we go back to the original with our savory, no-sugar-added, Paleo-perfected sloppy goodness.

1 medium onion

2 medium celery stalks

1 tablespoon avocado oil or bacon fat

1 teaspoon sea salt

1 pound ground beef

1 teaspoon garlic powder

1 teaspoon chili powder

1 (15-ounce) can tomato sauce

1 teaspoon Dijon mustard

4 to 8 large leaves of romaine lettuce, stemmed chard or kale, or cabbage

1. Chop the onion and celery.

2. In a large pan, heat the oil over medium heat. Add the onion, celery, and salt and cook, stirring, until crisp-tender, 3 to 5 minutes.

3. Add the ground beef, garlic powder, and chili powder to the pan with the veggies and cook, stirring occasionally, until almost browned, about 5 minutes. Stir in the tomato sauce and mustard, then reduce the heat to maintain a simmer and cook until the beef is cooked through, and the sauce is hot, about 5 minutes. Remove from the heat.

4. Portion ½ to 1 cup of the beef mixture onto each lettuce leaf, depending on how sloppy you want them. Double up the leaves, if needed.

Ingredient Tip: Use tomato sauce that doesn't contain any added sugar and comes in a BPA-free can or Tetra Pak. We like Muir Glen organic tomato sauce.

....

Per Serving (1 cup sauce and 2 lettuce leaves): Calories: 298; Total Fat: 18g; Protein: 24g; Carbohydrates: 10g; Fiber: 3g

"Spaghetti" and Meatballs

Egg-Free, Nut-Free
Serves 4 / Prep time: 5 minutes **/ Cook time:** 20 minutes

Spaghetti squash is the perfect pasta substitute. It's low-carb, looks like spaghetti, and tastes great. You can substitute ground turkey, ground chicken, or any other ground meat.

1 (3-pound) spaghetti squash
1 (25-ounce) jar marinara sauce (3 cups)
1 pound ground beef
1 tablespoon Italian seasoning
1 teaspoon sea salt
½ teaspoon garlic powder
½ teaspoon onion powder

1. Preheat the oven to 350°F. Line a rimmed baking sheet with parchment paper.

2. Fill a microwave-safe dish with ¼ to ½ inch of water. Cut the squash in half crosswise and scoop out the seeds. Place the squash cut-side down in the dish. Microwave on high for 15 minutes, or until the squash strands are tender. Let rest until cool enough to handle.

3. In a medium pot, heat the marinara over very low heat, stirring occasionally. In a large bowl, combine the ground beef, Italian seasoning, salt, garlic powder, and onion powder. Form the meat mixture into 12 balls and place on the prepared baking sheet. Bake for 20 to 25 minutes, until the meatballs are cooked through. Remove from the oven and transfer to the pot with the sauce. Stir to coat.

4. Using a fork, remove the squash strands from the shells. Top the spaghetti squash with the meatballs and sauce.

Technique Tip: To bake spaghetti squash, pierce several small holes in the shell. Place the whole squash in an oven-safe dish. Bake at 375°F for 60 minutes, or until easily pierced with a fork.

Per Serving (1 cup spaghetti squash, ¾ cup sauce, and 3 meatballs): Calories: 403; Total Fat: 24g; Protein: 23g; Carbohydrates: 26g; Fiber: 6g

Pepper Steak with Cilantro Rice

Egg-Free, Nut-Free
Serves 4 / Prep time: 20 minutes / **Cook time:** 10 minutes

You don't have to marinate beef overnight to impart fabulous flavor. A simple, quick marinade while you're prepping the rest of the meal is all it takes to produce mouthwatering taste. To save time, buy cauliflower that's already been riced, which is now widely available in markets. Grated ginger and minced garlic are also available in markets and are handy to keep in your refrigerator or freezer.

FOR THE MARINADE
¼ cup coconut aminos
2 tablespoons apple
   cider vinegar

FOR THE PEPPER STEAK
1 pound sirloin, flank
   steak, or strip steak
1 medium yellow onion,
   sliced
2 bell peppers, sliced
2 tablespoons
   avocado oil
1 tablespoon grated
   fresh ginger
2 garlic cloves, minced

1. **Make the marinade:** In a large bowl, combine the coconut aminos and vinegar.

2. **Prepare the pepper steak:** Thinly slice the steak into ¼-inch-thick strips. Add the steak to the bowl with the marinade and set aside for 15 minutes. Meanwhile, slice the onion and bell peppers.

3. **Make the cilantro rice:** If using a head of cauliflower, break it into florets and put in a food processor. Pulse several times, until the cauliflower resembles grains of rice. (Alternatively, finely dice the cauliflower by hand or grate on the large holes of a box grater.)

FOR THE CILANTRO RICE

1 large head
   cauliflower, or 4 cups
   riced cauliflower (see
   tip on page 46)
1 tablespoon
   avocado oil
1 garlic clove, minced
½ teaspoon sea salt
½ cup chopped fresh
   cilantro
2 scallions, chopped,
   for garnish

4. In a large pan, heat the oil over medium heat. Add the garlic and cook, stirring, for 1 minute. Add the riced cauliflower and salt and cook, stirring occasionally, until tender, about 3 minutes. Stir in the cilantro and cook for 1 minute more. Remove the cauliflower rice from the pan and set aside.

5. In the same pan, heat the oil over medium-high heat. Add the onion, peppers, ginger, and garlic and cook, stirring, for 2 minutes. Add the steak and cook, stirring frequently, for 2 to 3 minutes for medium doneness, or until the meat is cooked to your liking.

6. Enjoy the pepper steak alongside the cilantro rice, garnished with the scallions.

Switch It Up: Make this recipe AIP-friendly by swapping mushrooms or asparagus for the bell peppers.

Per Serving (4 ounces steak and veggies, and 1 cup rice): Calories: 372; Total Fat: 23g; Protein: 26g; Carbohydrates: 13g; Fiber: 4g

Perfect Paleo Chili

Egg-Free, Nut-Free
Serves 4 / Prep time: 5 minutes / **Cook time:** 25 minutes

Perfect chili in less than 30 minutes? You got it! With minimal prep and a quick simmer, you can have a batch of warm, comfort food the whole family will love. Toss a couple of handfuls of greens, such as spinach, kale, or chard, into the pot for the last two minutes of cooking to add a splash of color and a boost of nutrition.

2 large bell peppers

1 small onion

3 garlic cloves

1 tablespoon avocado oil, bacon fat, or coconut oil

1 pound ground beef

1½ tablespoons chili powder

2 teaspoons ground cumin

1 teaspoon sea salt

½ teaspoon freshly ground black pepper

1 (28-ounce) can crushed fire-roasted tomatoes, with their juices

1. Chop the bell peppers and onion into large dice. Mince the garlic.

2. In a large pot, heat the oil over medium heat. Add the bell pepper, onion, and garlic and cook, stirring frequently for 2 to 3 minutes, until the peppers start to soften.

3. Add the ground beef, chili powder, cumin, salt, and pepper and cook, stirring occasionally, for 5 to 7 minutes, until the beef is mostly browned.

4. Add the tomatoes and their juices to the pot and simmer for 15 minutes. Serve hot.

Switch It Up: Garnish with sliced avocado or fresh cilantro for a pretty finish that also boosts flavor and nutrition.

....

Per Serving (2 cups): Calories: 390; Total Fat: 25g; Protein: 23g; Carbohydrates: 16g; Fiber: 7g

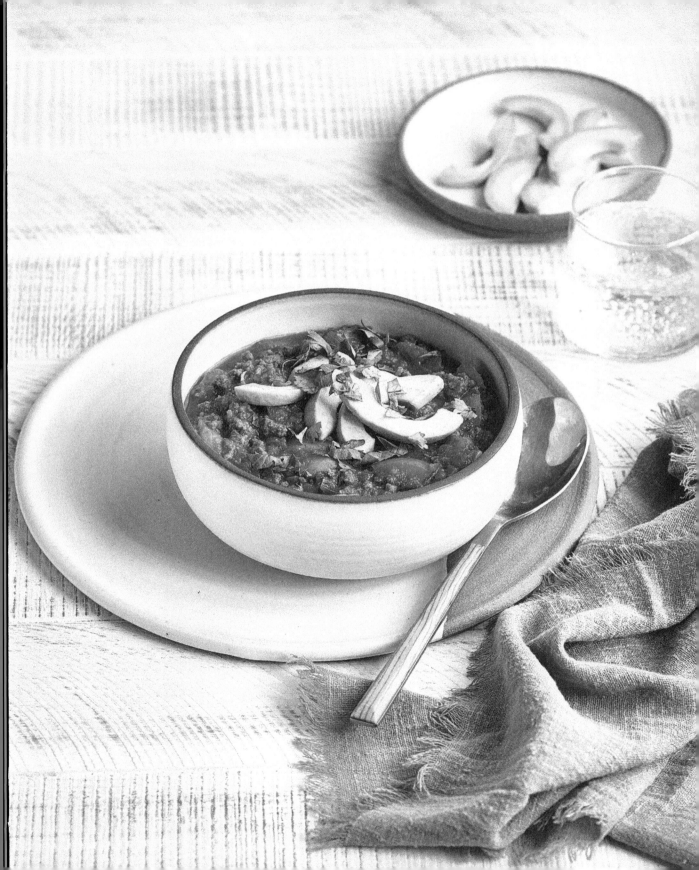

Pork Fried Rice

Nut-Free
Serves 4 / Prep time: 10 minutes **/ Cook time:** 15 minutes

You won't miss the takeout classic once you try this Paleo version. If you're not a fan of pork, swap in ground beef, lamb, chicken, or turkey.

1 tablespoon avocado oil

1 pound ground pork

1 large head cauliflower, or 4 cups riced cauliflower (see tip on page 46)

2 medium carrots

1 small onion

2 garlic cloves

1 tablespoon grated fresh ginger, or 1 teaspoon ground ginger

½ teaspoon sea salt

¼ teaspoon freshly ground black pepper

3 tablespoons coconut aminos

2 large eggs, beaten

2 tablespoons toasted sesame oil

2 medium scallions, chopped (optional)

1. In a large skillet, heat the oil over medium-high heat. Add the pork and cook, stirring occasionally, until browned, about 10 minutes. Remove the pork from the pan, leaving the fat behind, and set aside.

2. If using a head of cauliflower, break it into florets and put them in a food processor. Pulse several times, until the cauliflower resembles grains of rice, then transfer to a bowl. (Alternatively, finely dice the cauliflower by hand or grate on the large holes of a box grater.) Combine the carrots, onion, garlic, and ginger in the food processor and pulse until coarsely chopped (or chop by hand).

3. Add the carrots, onion, garlic, ginger, salt, and pepper to the fat left in the pan and cook over medium heat for 1 minute. Add the coconut aminos and riced cauliflower and cook, stirring occasionally, for 2 minutes.

4. Return the pork to the pan, add the eggs, and cook, stirring, until the pork is warm and the eggs are cooked through, about 3 minutes. Drizzle with the sesame oil, garnish with the scallions (if using) and serve.

Smart Shopping: To save time on this dish, purchase riced cauliflower, shredded carrots, chopped onions, and minced garlic and ginger.

....

Per Serving (1¾ cups): Calories: 314; Total Fat: 18g; Protein: 30g; Carbohydrates: 11g; Fiber: 4g

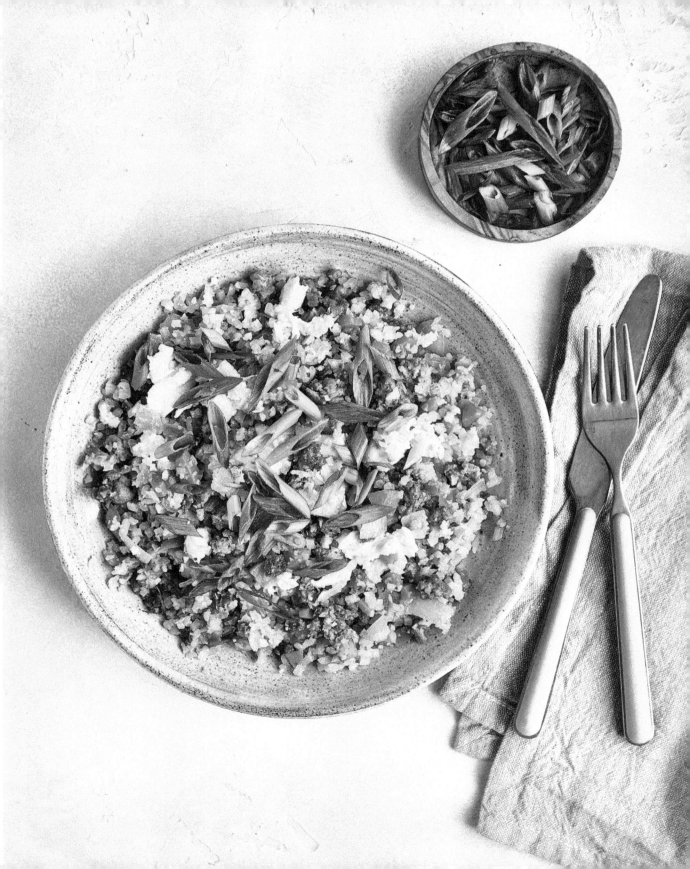

Steak with Mango Salsa

Egg-Free, Nut-Free
Serves 4 / Prep time: 10 minutes / **Cook time:** 10 minutes

Salsa is the Spanish word for "sauce." It is traditionally made with tomatoes and fresh chiles. These days, salsas are truly versatile—they can be savory, sweet, spicy, or mild. Here we use a sweet, fruity salsa that perfectly complements flank steak with its bright colors and flavors. You can cook your steak on the stovetop in a large pan over medium-high heat as an alternative to broiling it, if you prefer.

FOR THE BEEF
1 tablespoon
   avocado oil
1 teaspoon ground
   chipotle chile
1 teaspoon sea salt
1½ pounds flank steak

FOR THE MANGO SALSA
2 mangos, peeled and
   diced (2 cups)
1 bell pepper, diced
½ cup diced red onion
¼ cup chopped fresh
   cilantro
Juice of 1 lime
½ teaspoon sea salt

1. Preheat the broiler to high.

2. **Make the beef:** In a small bowl, mix the oil, chipotle, and salt. Rub the mixture all over both sides of the steak and place on a baking sheet.

3. Broil the steak for 4 to 6 minutes per side, until done to your liking. Remove from the oven and cover loosely with aluminum foil. Let rest for 10 minutes.

4. **Make the salsa:** While the steak is resting, in a medium bowl, combine the mangos, bell pepper, onion, cilantro, lime juice, and salt.

5. Slice the steak across the grain into ½-inch-thick slices. Serve with the mango salsa.

Switch It Up: If mangos aren't in season, you can use jarred or frozen mango or any seasonal fruit. We love apples in the fall and pears or kiwis in the winter.

Per Serving (6 ounces steak and 1 cup salsa): Calories: 441; Total Fat: 20g; Protein: 36g; Carbohydrates: 29g; Fiber: 4g

Breaded Pork Chops with Green Apple Slaw

Egg-Free
Serves 4 / Prep time: 10 minutes / **Cook time:** 15 minutes

Apples and pork pair perfectly. Green Granny Smith apples marry sweet and tart, a complementary contrast to savory pork, but feel free to use any type of apple you prefer.

FOR THE PORK CHOPS
1 cup almond flour
1 tablespoon Italian seasoning
1 teaspoon sea salt
4 (4- to 6-ounce) boneless or (8-ounce) bone-in pork chops
2 tablespoons avocado oil, bacon fat, or lard

FOR THE SLAW
½ head green cabbage
1 large green apple
¼ cup freshly squeezed lime juice (from 2 limes)
2 tablespoons avocado oil or extra-virgin olive oil
1 tablespoon apple cider vinegar
¼ teaspoon sea salt

1. **Make the pork chops:** Mix the almond flour, Italian seasoning, and salt together on a plate. Dredge the pork chops through the mixture to coat on both sides.

2. In a large pan, heat the oil over medium heat. Add the pork chops and cook for 7 to 8 minutes per side, until the juices run clear and the internal temperature reaches 145° to 150°F for medium-rare, 150° to 155°F for medium, and 155° to 160°F for medium-well.

3. **Make the slaw:** Thinly slice the cabbage and put in a large bowl. Core and thinly slice the apple and add it to the bowl. Add the lime juice, oil, vinegar, and salt and toss to combine.

4. Enjoy the pork chops with the slaw alongside.

Ingredient Tip: If you'd prefer to use all-purpose seasoning for the pork chops, you can make your own by mixing ½ teaspoon each of garlic powder, onion powder, dried oregano, dried rosemary, dried thyme, and ground black pepper.

Per Serving (1 pork chop and 1½ cups slaw): Calories: 366; Total Fat: 23g; Protein: 32g; Carbohydrates: 14g; Fiber: 4g

Lamb Kebabs with Paleo Hummus

Egg-Free, Nut-Free
Serves 4 / Prep time: 15 minutes / **Cook time:** 15 minutes

You can prepare these kebabs on skewers or deconstructed on a baking sheet. Either way, the juxtaposition of lamb, veggies, and hummus in this dish will have your mouth watering.

2 zucchini
½ small red onion
1 pound ground lamb
1 tablespoon finely
   chopped fresh
   rosemary, or
   1½ teaspoons dried
1 tablespoon apple
   cider vinegar
1¼ teaspoons sea salt,
   divided
¼ teaspoon freshly
   ground pepper
¼ teaspoon onion
   powder
1 pint cherry tomatoes
1 tablespoon
   extra-virgin olive oil
Paleo Hummus
   (page 150), optional

1. Preheat the oven to 375°F. Line a large rimmed baking sheet with parchment paper.

2. Cut the zucchini into ½-inch-thick rounds and the onion into 1-inch chunks.

3. In a medium bowl, combine the lamb, rosemary, vinegar, ¾ teaspoon of the salt, the pepper, and onion powder. Form the lamb mixture into 12 balls.

4. Using wooden or metal skewers, thread a meatball, followed by a piece of zucchini, two slices of onion, and a cherry tomato. Repeat so there are three meatballs per skewer and four skewers total. Brush the kebabs with the olive oil and season with the remaining ½ teaspoon salt. Bake for 15 to 20 minutes, until the meatballs are cooked through, and the veggies are soft.

5. While the kebabs are cooking, prepare the hummus. For an elegant presentation, place a few dollops of hummus in the center of a plate and rest the kebabs on top.

Love Your Leftovers: For a delicious snack, cut up veggies and use them as dippers for any leftover hummus.

....

Per Serving (1 kebab and ½ cup hummus): Calories: 545; Total Fat: 40g; Protein: 34g; Carbohydrates: 14g; Fiber: 4g

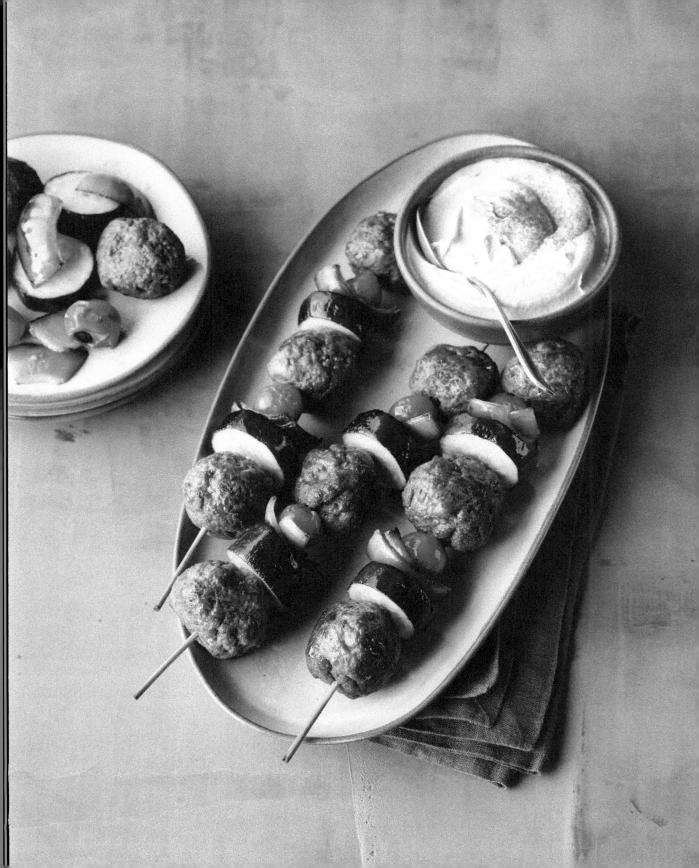

Rosemary Lamb Chops with Olive Tapenade and Green Beans

Egg-Free, Nut-Free
Serves 4 / Prep time: 10 minutes / **Cook time:** 15 minutes

Tapenade is a chunky, salty spread that wears many culinary hats. You can eat it alone as a snack, spread it on Paleo crackers, scoop it up with veggies, or use it to jazz up a meal of savory meat as we've done here.

FOR THE GREEN BEANS

12 ounces green beans, trimmed (about 2½ cups)

½ teaspoon sea salt

FOR THE OLIVE TAPENADE

1 cup pitted kalamata olives

1 cup pitted green olives

¼ cup fresh parsley

¼ cup fresh basil

2 garlic cloves

2 tablespoons extra-virgin olive oil

Juice of ½ lemon

FOR THE LAMB CHOPS

2 tablespoons avocado oil

2 pounds lamb chops

1 tablespoon dried rosemary

1 teaspoon sea salt

1. **Make the green beans:** Place a steamer basket in a medium pot and add water to reach the bottom of the basket. Bring to a boil over high heat. Add the green beans, season with the salt, cover, and steam for about 5 minutes, until crisp-tender. Remove the green beans from the pot with tongs and set aside.

2. **Make the olive tapenade:** While the beans are cooking, in a food processor, combine the kalamata and green olives, parsley, basil, garlic, olive oil, and lemon juice and pulse until finely chopped.

3. **Make the lamb chops:** In a large pan, heat the avocado oil over medium heat. Season both sides of the lamb chops with the rosemary and salt. Add the chops to the pan and cook for about 5 minutes per side, until done to your liking. Remove from the pan and cover loosely with aluminum foil to keep warm.

4. Stir the green beans into the juices remaining in the pan and heat until warmed, about 1 minute.

5. Serve green beans alongside lamb chops topped with a dollop of tapenade.

....

Per Serving (8 ounces lamb chops, ⅓ cup tapenade, and 3 ounces green beans): Calories: 402; Total Fat: 22g; Protein: 26g; Carbohydrates: 3g; Fiber: 0g

Pulled Pork

Egg-Free, Nut-Free
Serves 6 to 8 / Prep time: 10 minutes / **Cook time:** 6 hours

You can prep this recipe hours to days ahead of time. Refrigerate the prepped ingredients in the slow cooker insert; when you're ready, simply pop it in the slow cooker, turn it on, and forget about it until you're ready to eat! Be sure to freeze any excess for future use.

4 celery stalks

4 carrots

4 parsnips

1 onion

4 garlic cloves

1 cup chicken broth or bone broth

1 tablespoon paprika

1 tablespoon chili powder

1 tablespoon sea salt

1 teaspoon ground cinnamon

1 teaspoon garlic powder

1 teaspoon ground cumin

1 teaspoon freshly ground black pepper

1 (3½- to 4½-pound) pork shoulder roast

1. Chop the celery, carrots, parsnips, and onion into ½-inch pieces. Chop the garlic. Place the veggies in the slow cooker. Add the broth.

2. In a small bowl, combine the paprika, chili powder, salt, cinnamon, garlic powder, cumin, and pepper.

3. If needed, cut the pork so it will fit in your slow cooker. Rub the spice mixture all over the pork and place it in the slow cooker on top of the veggies. Cover and cook on High for 6 to 7 hours or on Low for 8 to 10 hours.

4. Transfer the pork to a cutting board and shred with two forks. Moisten the meat with juices from the pot and serve with the veggies on the side.

Technique Tip: To cook the pork in the oven instead, coat it with the spice mixture as directed, then sear in a skillet on the stovetop on all sides. Place the veggies in a baking dish large enough to hold the pork, set the seared pork on top, and bake at 325°F for 3 to 4 hours. Shred the meat and serve as directed.

Per Serving (1¼ cups pork and 1 cup vegetables): Calories: 547; Total Fat: 23g; Protein: 58g; Carbohydrates: 25g; Fiber: 7g

BLT Boats

Nut-Free
Serves 2 / Prep time: 5 minutes **/ Cook time:** 10 minutes

Just because you're Paleo doesn't mean you can't enjoy a good ol' bacon, lettuce, and tomato sandwich! This classic is wonderful as a wrap or chopped as a salad. Feel free to add any of your Paleo favorites: sliced onions, pickle spears, or deli meat like turkey or roast beef. These boats are a fantastic opportunity to eat gut-healing fermented raw veggies in the form of sauerkraut or kimchi.

8 bacon slices
2 large tomatoes
1 medium avocado
8 Bibb or Boston
   lettuce leaves
¼ cup Paleo
   mayonnaise

1. In a large pan, cook the bacon over medium-high heat, flipping the slices occasionally, until crispy, about 10 minutes. Transfer to a paper towel–lined plate and set aside.

2. While the bacon is cooking, cut the tomatoes and avocado into ¼-inch-thick slices.

3. Arrange the lettuce leaves in 4 stacks of 2 leaves each. Spread each wrap with 1 tablespoon of the mayonnaise, then layer with 2 slices of bacon, one-quarter of the tomatoes, and one-quarter of the avocado. Enjoy!

Ingredient Tip: To save yourself prep time and make this a superfast throw-together meal, buy cooked bacon and just crisp it in the microwave for a few seconds before serving.

....

Per Serving (2 wraps): Calories: 488; Total Fat: 38g; Protein: 20g; Carbohydrates: 20g; Fiber: 10g

Southwest Chorizo Stew

Egg-Free, Nut-Free
Serves 4 / Prep time: 10 minutes / **Cook time:** 25 minutes

Chorizo is the star of this Paleo stew. There are two types: cured Spanish chorizo, which is seasoned with smoked paprika and sold in links, and fresh Mexican chorizo, which is sold in casings or loose. Try topping each bowl with sliced avocado, chopped tomato, and sprigs of fresh cilantro.

1 large onion

1 large carrot

1 large celery stalk

1 bell pepper

1 large tomato

2 medium sweet potatoes

2 garlic cloves, peeled

1 pound cured Spanish chorizo or fresh Mexican chorizo

1 tablespoon avocado oil, coconut oil, or bacon fat

3 cups chicken broth or bone broth

1 tablespoon freshly squeezed lemon juice (from ½ lemon)

Pinch sea salt

Pinch freshly ground black pepper

1. Chop the onion, carrot, celery, bell pepper, tomato, and sweet potatoes into large dice. Mince the garlic. If using Spanish chorizo, slice it into ½-inch-thick pieces. If using Mexican chorizo in links, remove the meat from the casings.

2. In a large pot, heat the oil over medium-high heat. Add the onion, carrot, celery, bell pepper, and chorizo. Cook, stirring occasionally, until the chorizo starts to brown and the veggies start to soften, about 3 minutes. Keep in mind that Mexican chorizo will need a few extra minutes of cooking time. Remove all but 2 tablespoons of the rendered fat from the pot. Add the tomato, sweet potatoes, garlic, broth, and lemon juice. Cover and bring to a boil.

3. Reduce the heat to medium-low, cover, and simmer for 20 minutes, or until the potatoes are easily pierced with a fork.

4. Season with the salt and pepper, and serve.

Switch It Up: Any variety of sausage will be a perfect substitute for the chorizo—especially Italian or andouille sausages.

....

Per Serving (1½ cups): Calories: 495; Total Fat: 33g; Protein: 24g; Carbohydrates: 22g; Fiber: 4g

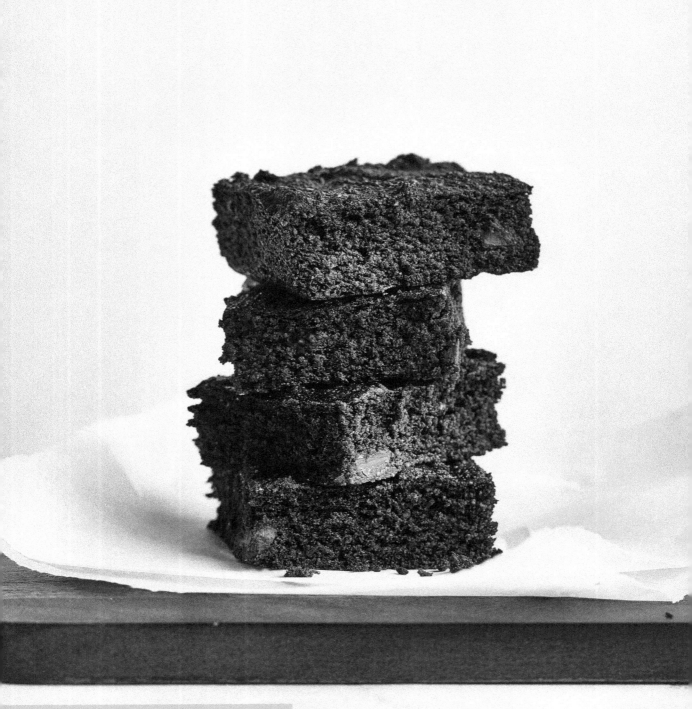

CHAPTER 8
Snacks and Desserts

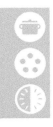

Sweet-and-Salty Bacon-Wrapped Dates

Egg-Free
Serves 6 / Prep time: 10 minutes **/ Cook time:** 10 minutes

Looking for a sweet, salty, crunchy all-in-one bite? We've got you covered with this amazing and simple recipe. Medjool dates impart a lovely natural sweetness that provides a striking contrast to salty bacon and crunchy almonds. Serve them as an appetizer or keep some in your refrigerator as a pick-me-up snack. Keep in mind that the carbs in dates add up quickly, so try to limit yourself to two at a time.

6 bacon slices
12 Medjool dates
12 whole almonds

1. Preheat the oven to 450°F. Place a wire rack on a rimmed baking sheet.

2. Cut each piece of bacon in half. Set aside.

3. With a paring knife, slice each date lengthwise through the center, being careful not to cut all the way through, and remove the pit. Place an almond in the center of each date, press the date back together to enclose the almond, and wrap with a piece of bacon. Place the bacon-wrapped dates on the rack, seam-side down.

4. Bake the dates for about 10 minutes, until the bacon is crispy or cooked to your liking, flipping them once during cooking. With tongs, transfer the dates to a paper towel–lined plate. Enjoy warm or at room temperature.

Switch It Up: When it comes to nuts, any variety will work in this recipe. We especially like using pecan halves or cashews instead of almonds.

Per Serving (2 dates): Calories: 186; Total Fat: 5g; Protein: 4g; Carbohydrates: 37g; Fiber: 4g

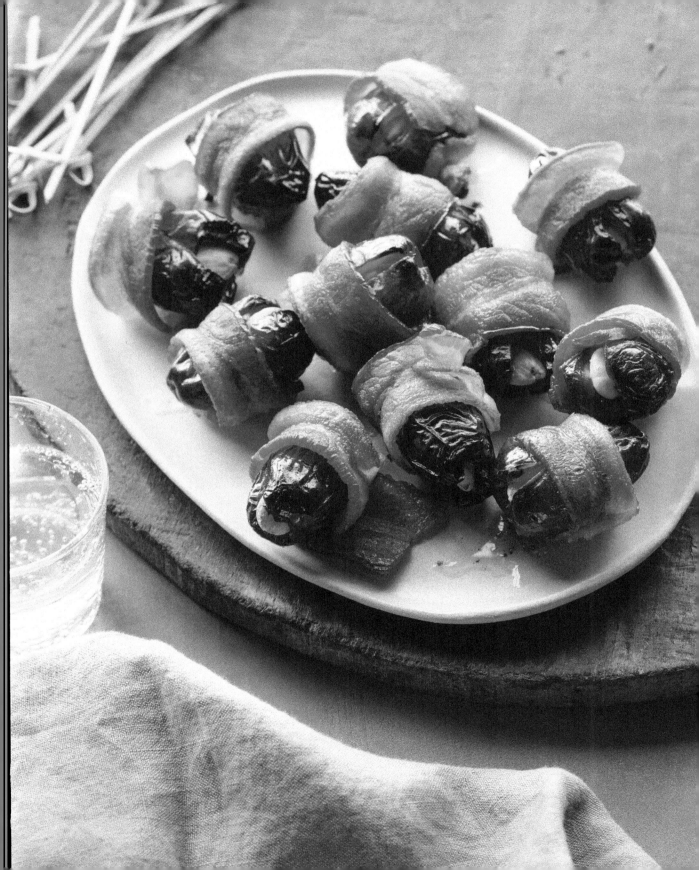

Paleo Pigs in a Blanket

Serves 8 / Prep time: 20 minutes **/ Cook time:** 20 minutes

These healthy pigs in a blanket are made with miniature smoked pork sausages, also called cocktail sausages or little smokies. Choose a brand that is uncured, nitrate-free, and fully cooked. You can make your own by cutting up grass-fed hot dogs.

1½ cups almond flour
½ cup tapioca flour or arrowroot flour
½ teaspoon sea salt
¼ teaspoon baking soda
1 large egg
2 tablespoons water
1 tablespoon ghee or coconut oil, melted
24 miniature smoked pork sausages, or 8 hot dogs

1. Preheat the oven to 350°F.

2. In a medium bowl, combine the almond flour, tapioca flour, salt, and baking soda. In a small bowl, whisk together the egg, water, and melted ghee. Pour the wet ingredients into the dry ingredients. Mix until the dough comes together and forms a ball.

3. Turn the dough out onto a cutting board. Cover with a piece of parchment paper the size of your baking sheet. Roll out the dough until you have a flat sheet about ⅛ inch thick. Place the parchment on the baking sheet and set aside. Cut the dough into 24 squares measuring roughly 1½ by 3 inches.

4. Pat the sausages dry. (If using hotdogs, cut them into 2-inch-long pieces.) Wrap a dough square around each sausage, leaving the ends uncovered. Place seam-side down, an inch apart, on the prepared baking sheet.

5. Bake for 20 to 25 minutes, until the dough turns a golden color.

Switch It Up: Add pizzazz to your dough by mixing 1 tablespoon Italian seasoning or garlic powder into the dry ingredients.

Per Serving (3 wrapped sausages): Calories: 262; Total Fat: 20g; Protein: 12g; Carbohydrates: 11g; Fiber: 2g

Happy Trails Mix

No-Cook, Vegan, Egg-Free
Makes 5 cups / Prep time: 5 minutes

Trail mix is one of the easiest ways to keep your snacks both Paleo and grab-and-go. There's no right or wrong way to do it—just throw together a batch with your favorite nuts, seeds, and dried fruit. We've added some dark chocolate chips for a little extra zip. Make sure your chocolate chips are Paleo-friendly and don't contain unwanted ingredients like soy or vegetable oils. Our favorite brand is Enjoy Life dark chocolate morsels.

1 cup raw almonds

1 cup raw cashews

1 cup raw macadamia nuts

½ cup hulled sunflower seeds

½ cup raw pumpkin seeds

½ cup raisins

¼ cup dark chocolate chips

1. In a medium bowl, combine the almonds, cashews, macadamia nuts, sunflower seeds, pumpkin seeds, raisins, and chocolate chips.

2. Store in individual serving containers for an easy grab-and-go snack or in an airtight container in a cool, dry place for up to several months.

Switch It Up: To reduce the added sugar content, omit the dark chocolate chips, or use 100% cacao dark chocolate chips. We like Pasha organic cacao chips.

Per Serving (½ cup): Calories: 370; Total Fat: 27g; Protein: 14g; Carbohydrates: 29g; Fiber: 5g

Paleo Hummus

Vegan, Egg-Free, Nut-Free
Serves 4 / Prep time: 10 minutes **/ Cook time:** 10 minutes

Hummus is a Middle Eastern dip traditionally made with chickpeas. Paleo hummus is made with cauliflower instead, but tastes remarkably like the original. This Paleo-friendly hummus is such a palate-pleaser, you'll find yourself making it over and over again. Enhance this recipe with a few tablespoons of chopped fresh dill or rosemary. Serve with your favorite crudités or grain-free crackers.

2 tablespoons extra-virgin olive oil
4 cups riced cauliflower (see tip on page 46)
2 teaspoons ground cumin
½ cup tahini
3 garlic cloves
Juice of 1 lemon
½ teaspoon sea salt
¼ teaspoon paprika, for garnish

1. In a large pan, heat the oil over medium heat. Add the riced cauliflower and cumin. Cook, stirring occasionally, until the cauliflower is soft, about 10 minutes.

2. Combine the tahini, garlic, lemon juice, and salt in a food processor or high-speed blender. Add the cooked cauliflower and process until smooth, about 1 minute, scraping down the sides with a rubber spatula as needed.

3. Transfer to a serving bowl, garnish with the paprika, and serve warm or cold.

....

Per Serving (½ cup): Calories: 300; Total Fat: 25g; Protein: 10g; Carbohydrates: 9g; Fiber: 3g

"Cheesy" Kale Chips

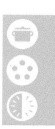

Vegan, AIP, Egg-Free, Nut-Free
Serves 4 / Prep time: 5 minutes **/ Cook time:** 20 minutes

Kale chips are a superhealthy crunchy snack that, once experienced, are sure to become a staple in your Paleo recipe repertoire. The "cheese" flavor comes from nutritional yeast, which is high in B vitamins and has a nutty flavor that is surprisingly reminiscent of real cheese.

8 cups packed
  stemmed curly kale
  leaves, torn into 2- to
  3-inch pieces
2 tablespoons
  avocado oil
¼ cup nutritional yeast
¼ teaspoon sea salt

1. Preheat the oven to 325°F.

2. Combine the kale, oil, nutritional yeast, and salt in a large bowl and, using your hands, toss to completely coat the kale.

3. Spread the kale in a single layer over a rimmed baking sheet and bake until the kale is crispy, 20 to 25 minutes.

4. Enjoy as a snack or as a side dish to your favorite Paleo entrée.

Switch It Up: Enhance the flavor profile of your kale with additional seasonings. For instance, try adding a few teaspoons of curry powder, garlic powder, or onion powder in step 2.

Per Serving (1 cup): Calories: 105; Total Fat: 7g; Protein: 4g; Carbohydrates: 6g; Fiber: 2g

Paleo Party Nachos

Egg-Free, Nut-Free
Serves 6 / Prep time: 10 minutes **/ Cook time:** 10 minutes

Nachos are a party favorite, and they make a great high-protein snack, too. Instead of corn tortilla chips, we've used Paleo-friendly plantain chips. These sturdy chips hold up well under the meat and fixings. Siete Foods grain-free tortilla chips is another excellent option.

1½ teaspoons chili powder

1½ teaspoons ground cumin

1½ teaspoons garlic powder

1 teaspoon onion powder

½ teaspoon sea salt

¼ teaspoon freshly ground black pepper

¼ teaspoon cayenne pepper (optional)

1 pound ground beef

1 (4-ounce) can green chiles, undrained

3 cups plantain chips

1 cup salsa

½ cup guacamole, homemade (see page 162) or store-bought

2 jalapeños, sliced (optional)

½ cup chopped fresh cilantro, for garnish (optional)

1. In a small bowl, combine the chili powder, cumin, garlic powder, onion powder, salt, pepper, and cayenne (if using).

2. In a large pan, combine the ground beef with the seasoning mix and cook over medium-high heat until the meat is almost browned, about 6 minutes. Add the green chiles and their liquid and cook for 1 to 2 minutes more, until the meat is fully cooked and the chiles are warmed through.

3. Arrange the plantain chips on a large platter. Layer the meat, salsa, and guacamole over the chips. Top with the jalapeños and cilantro, if desired, and serve.

Switch It Up: Use any ground meat that you have on hand, such as ground chicken, turkey, lamb, or even something more exotic like bison.

....

Per Serving (½ cup chips plus ½ cup meat and toppings): Calories: 379; Total Fat: 22g; Protein: 16g; Carbohydrates: 30g; Fiber: 2g

Raspberry Almond Muffins

Vegetarian
Makes 12 muffins / Prep time: 10 minutes **/ Cook time:** 20 minutes

These muffins might as well be called cupcakes, except they are made with only wholesome Paleo ingredients. This recipe is versatile, and any type of berry or flavoring will work. Try swapping blueberries for the raspberries and vanilla for the almond extract. This recipe is super easy to make in a food processor. Simply mix all the ingredients together, bake, and enjoy . . . guilt-free!

3 large eggs
⅓ cup maple syrup
⅓ cup melted coconut oil or ghee
1 teaspoon almond extract
2 cups almond flour
½ cup tapioca flour or arrowroot flour
½ teaspoon baking soda
¼ teaspoon sea salt
1 cup fresh raspberries

1. Preheat the oven to 350°F. Line a 12-cup muffin tin with paper liners if not using silicone baking cups.

2. Combine the eggs, maple syrup, melted coconut oil, and almond extract in a food processor. Process until combined. (Alternatively, mix by hand in a medium bowl using a large spoon.)

3. Add the almond flour, tapioca flour, baking soda, and salt to the food processor or bowl with the wet ingredients and mix until thoroughly combined. Gently stir the raspberries into the batter. Divide the batter evenly among the prepared muffin cups.

4. Bake for 20 to 25 minutes, until the muffins are lightly golden on top and a toothpick inserted into the center of a muffin comes out mostly clean.

Switch It Up: To make a delicious crumble topping, mix ¼ cup coconut sugar with 1 tablespoon each of almond flour, tapioca flour or arrowroot flour, and melted coconut oil. Sprinkle the topping over the muffins before baking.

Per Serving (1 muffin): Calories: 208; Total Fat: 15g; Protein: 5g; Carbohydrates: 15g; Fiber: 3g

Guilt-Free Brownies

Vegetarian, Nut-Free
Makes 9 brownies / Prep time: 5 minutes / **Cook time:** 25 minutes

Grain-free means guilt-free, and these brownies are both. Decadent and delicious, these easy blender brownies satisfy when a chocolate craving hits. Your Paleo diet should never be centered around sweets, but an occasional indulgence won't set you back one bit. Blending the eggs on high speed for 1 to 3 minutes helps the brownies rise beautifully.

3 large eggs
1 large avocado
¾ cup pure maple syrup
¼ cup unsweetened applesauce
1 tablespoon freshly squeezed lemon juice (from ½ lemon)
1 tablespoon pure vanilla extract
½ cup coconut flour
½ cup unsweetened cacao or cocoa powder
1 teaspoon baking soda
½ teaspoon sea salt
¼ cup dark chocolate chips or cacao chips

1. Preheat the oven to 325°F. Line the bottom of an 8-inch square baking pan with a piece of parchment paper cut to fit.

2. In a blender or food processor, blend the eggs on high for 1 to 3 minutes. Add the avocado, maple syrup, applesauce, lemon juice, and vanilla and blend until smooth. Add the coconut flour, cacao powder, baking soda, and salt and pulse until well combined. Stir in the chocolate chips by hand or gently pulse them in. Spoon the batter into the prepared pan and spread it evenly.

3. Bake for 25 to 30 minutes, until set and cooked through. Let cool in the pan before cutting into nine squares and enjoying.

Switch It Up: For a nutty brownie, add ¼ cup chopped walnuts or nut of choice.

....

Per Serving (1 brownie): Calories: 187; Total Fat: 9g; Protein: 4g; Carbohydrates: 26g; Fiber: 4g

Choose Your Own Cookie Adventure

Vegan, Egg-Free
Makes 24 cookies / Prep time: 10 minutes **/ Cook time:** 10 minutes

Miss cookies? No longer! This recipe provides the base for a number of different cookie types, so you can choose your own cookie adventure. Try subbing in almond extract for the vanilla or sprinkling cinnamon into the mix. The possibilities are quite endless.

½ cup avocado oil
    or melted ghee or
    coconut oil
½ cup pure maple syrup
1 tablespoon pure
    vanilla extract
2 cups almond flour
2 tablespoons coconut
    flour
½ teaspoon baking
    soda
½ teaspoon sea salt
½ cup cookie add-ins
    (chocolate chips,
    cacao chips, chopped
    nuts, dried fruit,
    coconut flakes, etc.)

1. In a food processor, combine the oil, maple syrup, and vanilla and pulse until combined. Add the almond flour, coconut flour, baking soda, and salt and process until combined. Pulse or stir in the add-ins. (Alternatively, make the dough in a large bowl, stirring by hand with a large spoon.) Cover the dough and refrigerate for at least 30 minutes.

2. Preheat the oven to 350°F. Line two large baking sheets with parchment paper.

3. Spoon heaping tablespoons of dough about 2 inches apart onto the prepared baking sheets.

4. Bake for 10 to 15 minutes, depending on how crispy you like your cookies. Let cool on the baking sheets for at least 10 minutes to finish setting before enjoying.

Ingredient Tip: For the best results, use blanched almond flour in this recipe.

Per Serving (2 cookies): Calories: 248; Total Fat: 20g; Protein: 4g; Carbohydrates: 16g; Fiber: 3g

Fall Flavors Granola

Vegan
Makes 4 cups / Prep time: 10 minutes **/ Cook time:** 15 minutes

Enjoy this granola as a snack, on coconut yogurt, or doused in nut milk for a satisfying breakfast.

¼ cup pure maple syrup
¼ cup coconut oil
2 teaspoons pumpkin pie spice
Pinch sea salt
1 cup almonds
1 cup cashews
1 teaspoon pure vanilla extract
⅓ cup pumpkin seeds
⅓ cup hulled sunflower seeds
¼ cup unsweetened coconut flakes
¾ cup unsweetened dried blueberries, dried cherries, or raisins

1. Preheat the oven to 325°F. Line a rimmed baking sheet with parchment paper.

2. In a saucepan, combine the maple syrup, oil, pumpkin pie spice, and salt and heat over low heat, whisking occasionally, until warm, about 3 minutes.

3. Combine the almonds and cashews in a food processor. Pulse a few times to coarsely chop (do not overprocess into nut butter). Alternatively, use a knife to coarsely chop the nuts. Add the nuts, vanilla, pumpkin seeds, sunflower seeds, and coconut flakes to the saucepan and stir to coat them with the maple syrup mixture.

4. Pour the mixture onto the prepared baking sheet and spread it evenly. Bake the granola for 15 to 20 minutes, until lightly browned. Remove from the oven and add the dried blueberries, pressing them lightly into the granola. Let cool for 20 minutes.

5. Break the cooled granola into pieces with the spatula. Store in an airtight container at room temperature for up to 2 weeks.

Switch It Up: Any type of nut will work in this recipe.

Per Serving (½ cup): Calories: 385; Total Fat: 28g; Protein: 13g; Carbohydrates: 27g; Fiber: 5g

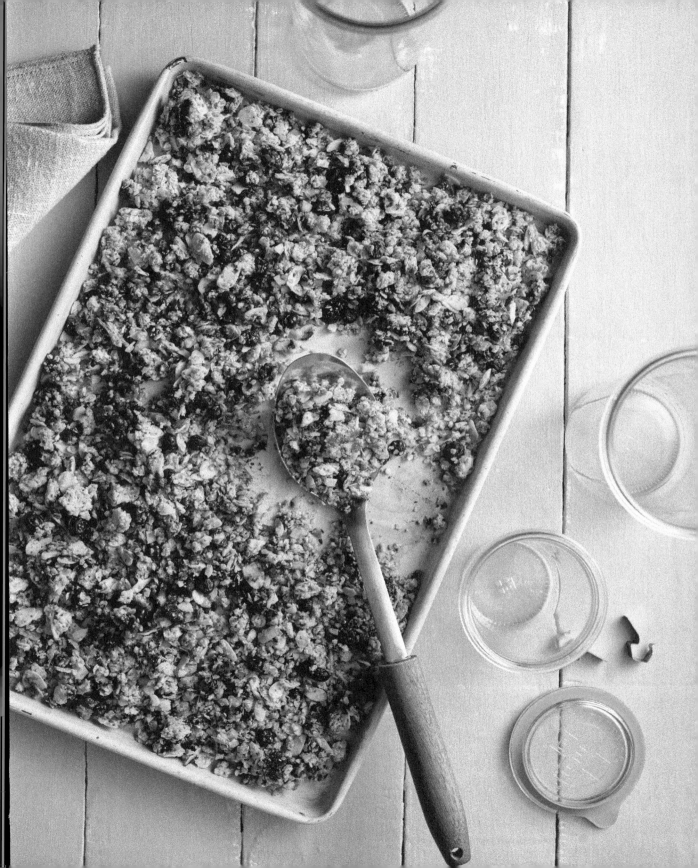

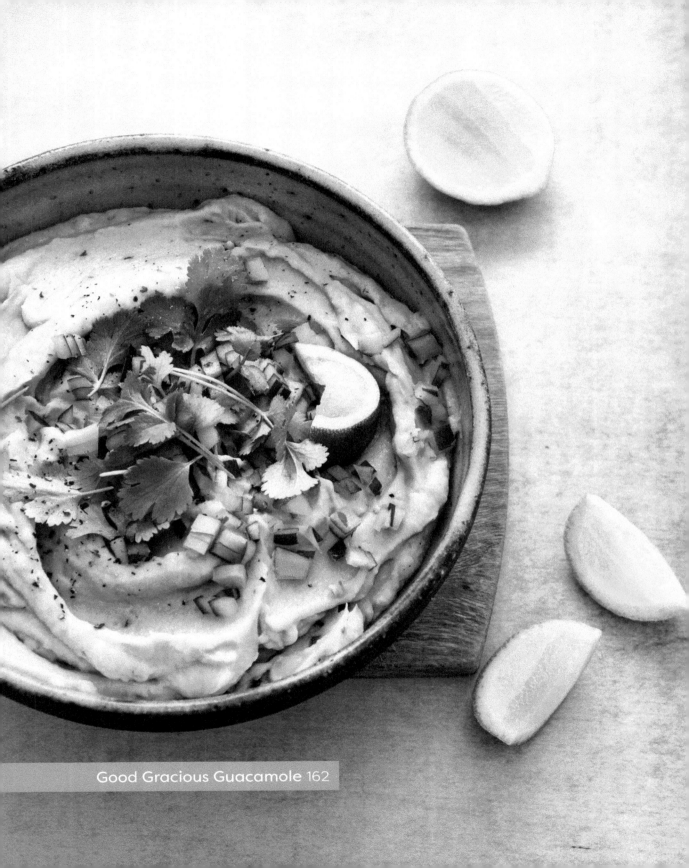

Good Gracious Guacamole 162

CHAPTER 9

Homemade Staples

Paleo Tortillas

Vegetarian, Nut-Free
Makes 8 tortillas / Prep time: 5 minutes **/ Cook time:** 25 minutes

This recipe upgrades traditional tortillas, replacing grain flours with coconut and tapioca flours. Fry them long enough to achieve a crisp taco shell, and no longer will you mourn tortillas on your Paleo diet!

2 large eggs
1 cup full-fat coconut milk
2 tablespoons avocado oil, divided, plus more if needed
1 cup tapioca flour
¼ cup coconut flour
¼ teaspoon sea salt

1. In a medium bowl, whisk the eggs. Add the coconut milk and 1 tablespoon of the oil and whisk until well combined.

2. In a large bowl, mix the tapioca flour, coconut flour, and salt.

3. Pour the wet ingredients into the dry ingredients and stir until fully combined.

4. In a large skillet, heat the remaining 1 tablespoon oil over medium heat. When hot, pour a scant ¼ cup of the batter into the center of the skillet and use a spoon to spread the batter or quickly rotate the pan, forming a 6-inch circle. Cook for 1 to 2 minutes, until the tortilla is firm enough to flip. Use a spatula to flip and cook for 1 minute on the second side. Transfer to a paper towel–lined plate. Repeat with the remaining batter. You may need to add additional oil to the skillet halfway through the process.

5. Enjoy the tortillas filled with your favorite Paleo fixings.

Appliance Tip: For efficiency, put all ingredients in a food processor or blender and mix until combined.

....

Per Serving (1 tortilla): Calories: 162; Total Fat: 13g; Protein: 2g; Carbohydrates: 10g; Fiber: 1g

Grain-Free Sandwich Bread

Vegetarian
Makes 12 slices / Prep time: 5 minutes **/ Cook time:** 25 minutes

Transform this bread into avocado toast or a sandwich with your favorite Paleo fixings, or heat it in the oven with ghee and crushed garlic for delicious garlic bread. Use your imagination, because whatever conventional bread can do, Paleo bread can do better.

Avocado oil, ghee,
   or coconut oil, for
   greasing
3 cups almond flour
¾ cup arrowroot flour
   or tapioca flour
¾ teaspoon baking
   soda
¾ teaspoon sea salt
5 large eggs
1½ teaspoons apple
   cider vinegar

1. Preheat the oven to 350°F. Line the bottom of a 9-by-5-inch loaf pan with a piece of parchment paper cut to fit. Grease the parchment and the sides of the pan with avocado oil, ghee, or coconut oil.

2. In a medium bowl, combine the almond flour, arrowroot flour, baking soda, and salt.

3. In a large bowl, whisk the eggs until frothy, about 1 minute, then stir the vinegar into the eggs.

4. Add the dry ingredients to the wet and mix until just combined. (Alternatively, combine all dry and wet ingredients in a food processor.)

5. Pour the batter into the prepared pan. Bake for 25 to 30 minutes, until a toothpick inserted into the center comes out clean.

6. Turn the bread out of the pan and transfer to a wire rack to cool completely. Cut into 12 slices and serve, or store in an airtight container in the refrigerator for up to 5 days.

Per Serving (1 slice): Calories: 148; Total Fat: 9g; Protein: 6g; Carbohydrates: 10g; Fiber: 2g

Good Gracious Guacamole

No-Cook, Vegan, Egg-Free, Nut-Free
Serves 4 / Prep time: 10 minutes

Avocados are an incredibly nutritious fruit, full of 20 different vitamins and minerals, healthy fats, and anti-inflammatory compounds. The Hass avocado from Mexico is the most common type found in markets and used in recipes. Avocados can be baked, broiled, fried, cut into chunks for salad, sliced for sandwiches, or mashed for—you guessed it—guacamole. We listed our favorite toppings here, but feel free to add any others you like or omit them entirely.

2 large avocados
2 tablespoons minced fresh cilantro
2 teaspoons freshly squeezed lime juice (from ½ lime)
¼ teaspoon sea salt
1 to 2 tablespoons add-ins, such as minced fresh chives, minced red onion, sliced jalapeños, diced tomatoes, crumbled cooked bacon, pomegranate seeds, or diced jicama (optional)

1. Halve and pit the avocados, then scoop the flesh out of the skin into a medium bowl. Mash the avocado with a fork until no large lumps remain.

2. Add the cilantro, lime juice, and salt and mix to combine.

3. Enjoy immediately, topped with your favorite add-ins, if desired.

Ingredient Tip: Mashed avocado makes a great substitute for Paleo mayonnaise if you don't have any on hand. Use it in recipes in the same proportions as you would use mayo.

Per Serving (¼ cup): Calories: 108; Total Fat: 10g; Protein: 1g; Carbohydrates: 7g; Fiber: 5g

Paleo Mayonnaise

No-Cook, Vegetarian, Nut-Free
Makes 1 cup / Prep time: 10 minutes

Learning to make your own mayonnaise is a Paleo rite of passage. Luckily, this recipe is quick and easy and works every time. It takes all of 10 minutes to whip up a smooth, creamy, lemony homemade mayo that tastes so good, you're likely to swear off the store-bought stuff forever. Any healthy oil, including olive oil, avocado oil, and macadamia nut oil, will produce perfectly Paleo mayonnaise.

2 large egg yolks
2 tablespoons freshly squeezed lemon juice (from 1 lemon)
1 cup extra-virgin olive oil
1 teaspoon Dijon mustard
Pinch sea salt

1. In a medium bowl, combine the egg yolks and lemon juice. With a handheld mixer or an immersion blender, beat the yolks and lemon juice together for a few seconds. (Alternatively, whisk them together by hand; if you choose to do so, use brisk strokes.)

2. With the mixer or blender running (or while whisking continuously), very slowly add the oil in a thin drizzle and mix until the mixture is thickened and emulsified. It can take as long as 3 to 5 minutes to fully incorporate the oil, so be patient and don't pour too fast.

3. Once the mixture is opaque and resembles mayonnaise, blend in the mustard and salt. Use immediately or store in an airtight container in the refrigerator for up to 4 days.

Ingredient Tip: The risk of contracting salmonella from uncooked eggs is very small; however, you can use pasteurized eggs to further reduce the risk, if you prefer.

Per Serving (2 tablespoons): Calories: 275; Total Fat: 29g; Protein: 1g; Carbohydrates: 0g; Fiber: 0g

Tomato Ketchup

No-Cook, Vegan, Egg-Free, Nut-Free
Makes 1½ cups / Prep time: 5 minutes

Paleo ketchup can be used as a condiment or a sauce, and it's so yummy, you'll want to make enough to always have on hand. Slather it on burgers, steaks, and eggs, and use it as a dip for fries or even veggies. There are no refined sugars or additives here—just real ingredients for a naturally sweet-and-savory Paleo-friendly ketchup. Serve with Kickin' Chicken Strips (page 108) or Sweet Potato Fries (page 64).

2 (6-ounce) cans
    tomato paste
⅔ cup water
⅓ cup apple cider
    vinegar
1 teaspoon garlic
    powder
1 teaspoon onion
    powder
¾ teaspoon sea salt

Mix the ingredients. In a blender or by hand in a medium bowl, mix the tomato paste, water, vinegar, garlic powder, onion powder, and salt until well combined. Store in an airtight container in the refrigerator for up to 2 weeks. Enjoy with any of your favorite Paleo meals.

Switch It Up: Kick up the heat of your ketchup by adding cayenne, a couple of tablespoons of sriracha, or your favorite hot sauce to taste. Transform it into an amazing curry ketchup by adding 1 tablespoon curry powder.

Per Serving (2 tablespoons): Calories: 32g; Total Fat: 0g; Protein: 1g; Carbohydrates: 6g; Fiber: 2g

Whole Roasted Chicken

AIP, Egg-Free, Nut-Free
Serves 4 / Prep time: 5 minutes / **Cook time:** 1 hour

Roasting a whole chicken is one of the most useful cooking skills you can learn. And it's actually quite easy! Many recipes call for leftover cooked chicken or meat from a rotisserie chicken. This whole roasted chicken works wonderfully in soups, salads, stir-fries, or as a stand-alone meal. Cut it into pieces and freeze the leftovers for quick future use. Be sure to save the carcass and giblets to make Homemade Bone Broth (page 168).

1 tablespoon Italian seasoning

1 to 2 teaspoons sea salt

1 teaspoon freshly ground black pepper

1 (3- to 5-pound) whole chicken, giblets removed

1 tablespoon extra-virgin olive, avocado, or coconut oil

1. Adjust an oven rack to the middle position and preheat the oven to 375°F. Place a wire rack in a roasting pan or on a rimmed baking sheet.

2. In a small bowl, mix the Italian seasoning, salt, and pepper. Pat the chicken dry and rub the entire surface of its skin with the oil. Rub the oil underneath its skin as well, directly on the meat. Rub the seasoning mixture evenly over the outside of the bird. Place the chicken breast-side up on the rack. Tie the legs together with twine and tuck the wing tips behind the bird's back.

3. Roast for 15 to 20 minutes per pound, until a thermometer inserted into the thickest part of the thigh registers 165°F and the juices run clear when you cut between the leg and thigh.

Switch It Up: For more flavor, stuff the cavity of the bird with coarsely chopped onion, garlic cloves, fresh herbs, or sliced lemon.

....

Per Serving (4 ounces chicken with skin): Calories: 215; Total Fat: 12g; Protein: 25g; Carbohydrates: 0; Fiber: 0g

Paleo Ranch Dressing

No-Cook, Vegetarian, Nut-Free
Makes 1¾ cups / Prep time: 10 minutes

There are no processed ingredients in sight in this creamy blend of healthy fats and spices. Homemade ranch dressing is simple to prepare and sublime in its combination of flavors. By using your own mayo or an avocado oil–based store-bought variety, you avoid harmful inflammatory oils. Use Paleo ranch on salads or as a dip for Sweet Potato Fries (page 64) or your favorite Paleo dippers.

1 cup Paleo
  mayonnaise
¾ cup full-fat coconut
  milk
2 tablespoons finely
  chopped fresh
  parsley, or 1 teaspoon
  dried
2 tablespoons finely
  chopped fresh chives,
  or 1 teaspoon dried
1 teaspoon dried dill
1 teaspoon garlic
  powder
1 teaspoon onion
  powder
½ teaspoon sea salt
½ teaspoon freshly
  ground black pepper

Mix the ingredients. In a medium bowl, combine the mayonnaise, coconut milk, parsley, chives, dill, garlic powder, onion powder, salt, and pepper. Mix until smooth and creamy. Store in an airtight container in the refrigerator for up to 1 week.

Technique Tip: To transform this recipe into a thick ranch dip, use only ½ cup coconut milk and refrigerate before serving.

Per Serving (2 tablespoons): Calories: 131; Total Fat: 15g; Protein: 0g; Carbohydrates: 1g; Fiber: 0g

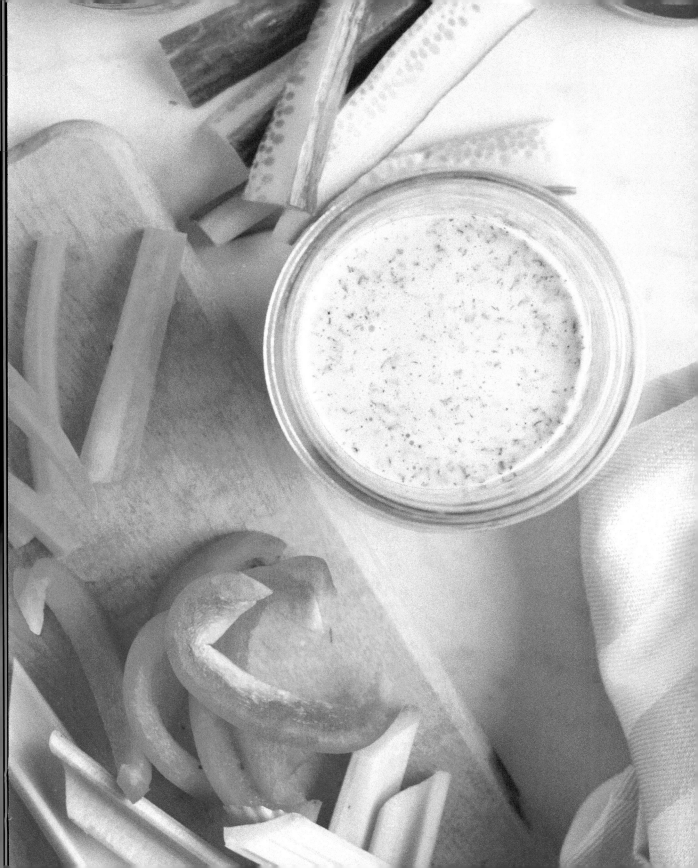

Homemade Bone Broth

AIP, Egg-Free, Nut-Free
Makes about 12 cups / Prep time: 30 minutes / **Cook time:** 5 hours

Broth made from the bones of any animal is full of collagen and gelatin, minerals, and amino acids such as glycine that are essential for gut health, proper immune function, and wound healing.

2 pounds beef, lamb, chicken, or turkey bones
2 large celery stalks
1 large carrot
1 large parsnip
1 large onion
1 cup chopped fresh parsley
2 tablespoons sea salt
2 tablespoons apple cider vinegar
1 tablespoon dried oregano
1 teaspoon dried thyme
3 bay leaves
12 cups water, plus more as needed

1. If you're using raw bones that aren't left over from previously roasted food, preheat the oven to 400°F (for chicken and turkey bones) or (450°F for beef and lamb bones). Line a baking sheet with parchment paper. Place the bones on the prepared baking sheet and roast for 20 minutes (for poultry) or 30 minutes (for beef and lamb). Remove the bones from the oven and transfer to a stockpot or other large pot.

2. Cut the celery, carrot, parsnip, and onion into large chunks and add them to the pot.

3. Add the parsley, salt, vinegar, oregano, thyme, bay leaves, and enough water to cover the contents of the pot. Bring to a boil over high heat, then reduce the heat to low, cover, and simmer for at least 5 hours and up to 24 hours, adding more water as needed to keep the solids covered.

4. Strain the broth through a fine-mesh strainer set over a large bowl. Transfer to an airtight container and store in the refrigerator for up to 4 days or in the freezer for up to 6 months.

Appliance Tip: You can make bone broth in your slow cooker. Combine the ingredients in the slow cooker, cover, and cook on low heat for at least 24 hours and up to 72 hours.

....

Per Serving (1 cup): Calories: 82; Total Fat: 7g; Protein: 9g; Carbohydrates: 2g; Fiber: 1g

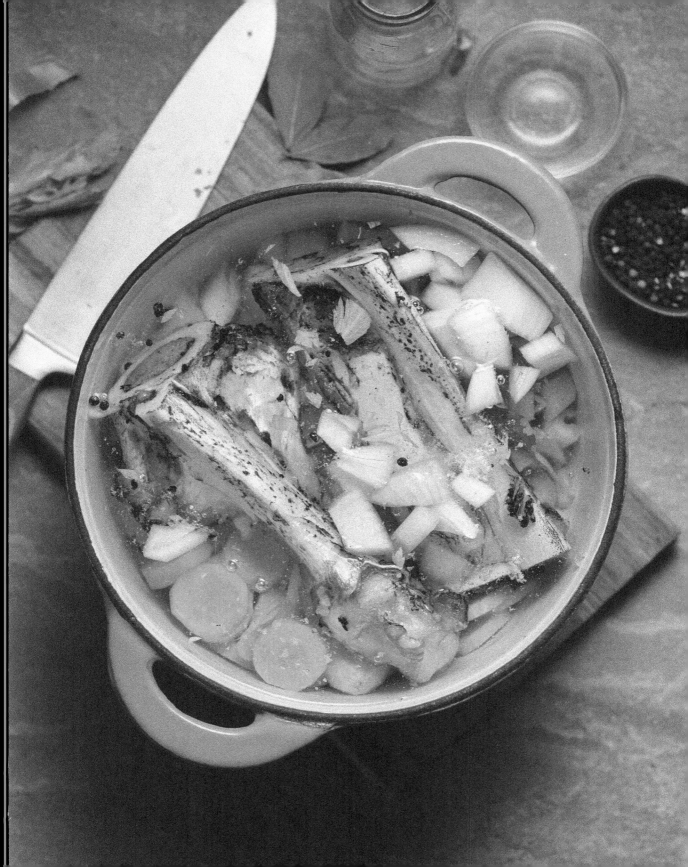

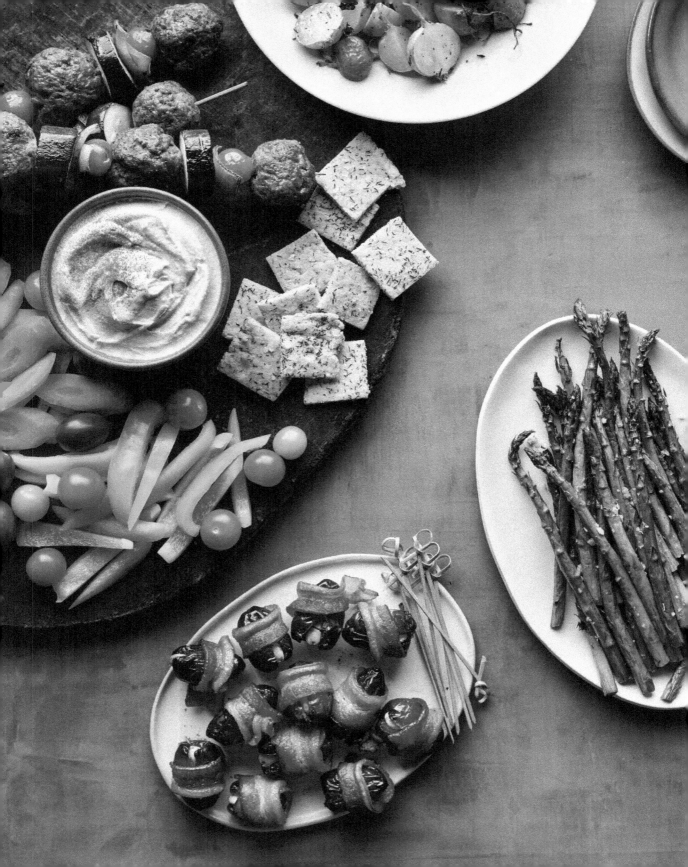

Measurement Conversions

VOLUME EQUIVALENTS

	U.S. STANDARD	U.S. STANDARD (OUNCES)	METRIC (APPROXIMATE)
LIQUID	2 tablespoons	1 fl. oz.	30 mL
	¼ cup	2 fl. oz.	60 mL
	½ cup	4 fl. oz.	120 mL
	1 cup	8 fl. oz.	240 mL
	1½ cups	12 fl. oz.	355 mL
	2 cups or 1 pint	16 fl. oz.	475 mL
	4 cups or 1 quart	32 fl. oz.	1 L
	1 gallon	128 fl. oz.	4 L
DRY	⅛ teaspoon	–	0.5 mL
	¼ teaspoon	–	1 mL
	½ teaspoon	–	2 mL
	¾ teaspoon	–	4 mL
	1 teaspoon	–	5 mL
	1 tablespoon	–	15 mL
	¼ cup	–	59 mL
	⅓ cup	–	79 mL
	½ cup	–	118 mL
	⅔ cup	–	156 mL
	¾ cup	–	177 mL
	1 cup	–	235 mL
	2 cups or 1 pint	–	475 mL
	3 cups	–	700 mL
	4 cups or 1 quart	–	1 L
	½ gallon	–	2 L
	1 gallon	–	4 L

OVEN TEMPERATURES

FAHRENHEIT	CELSIUS (APPROXIMATE)
250°F	120°C
300°F	150°C
325°F	165°C
350°F	180°C
375°F	190°C
400°F	200°C
425°F	220°C
450°F	230°C

WEIGHT EQUIVALENTS

U.S. STANDARD	METRIC (APPROXIMATE)
½ ounce	15 g
1 ounce	30 g
2 ounces	60 g
4 ounces	115 g
8 ounces	225 g
12 ounces	340 g
16 ounces or 1 pound	455 g

Resources

The following resources provide a wealth of science-backed, cutting-edge health information from the world's leading Paleo authorities.

The Paleo 30-Day Challenge cookbook by Kinsey Jackson and Sally Johnson is packed with 75 delicious recipes, four weeks of meal plans, and plenty of beginner-friendly information.

The Paleo Instant Pot Cookbook for Beginners by Kinsey Jackson and Sally Johnson contains 75 easy and mouthwatering recipes. Modern tools like the Instant Pot combined with an ancestral way of eating is a winning combination!

ChrisKresser.com offers evidence-based information and training. Chris is a leading authority in the fields of functional medicine and the Paleo diet.

The Environmental Working Group (EWG) is a nonprofit organization dedicated to environmental accountability. It publishes the Dirty Dozen, the Consumer Guide to Seafood, and other helpful resources.

MarksDailyApple.com presents research-based information and actionable tips for living a primal lifestyle in a modern world.

PaleoHacks.com contains a wealth of information on everything Paleo, including resources, books, and recipes to make living a Paleo lifestyle easy.

PaleoPlan.com offers customizable Paleo meal plans and hundreds of free recipes designed by a team of health experts.

RobbWolf.com is a best-selling author and expert providing science-based information about the Paleo and keto diets.

ThePaleoDiet.com provides books, research, and recipes by Dr. Loren Cordain, considered the modern-day founder of the Paleo diet.

ThePaleoMom.com is the website of Dr. Sarah Ballantyne, the foremost authority on the Paleo autoimmune protocol (AIP).

References

Cordain, Loren, et al. "Origins and Evolution of the Western Diet: Health Impli-cations for the 21st Century," *American Journal of Clinical Nutrition* 81, no. 2 (February 2005): 341–54, DOI: 10.1093/ajcn.81.2.341.

De Punder, Karin, and Leo Pruimboom. "The Dietary Intake of Wheat and Other Cereal Grains and Their Role in Inflammation," *Nutrients* 5, no. 3 (March 2013): 771–87, DOI: 10.3390/nu5030771.

Fasano, Alessio. "Zonulin and Its Regulation of Intestinal Barrier Function: The Biological Door to Inflammation, Autoimmunity, and Cancer," *Physiological Reviews* 91, no. 1 (January 2011): 151–75, DOI: 10.1152/physrev.00003.2008.

Ghaedi, Ehsan, Mohammad Mohammadi, Hamed Mohammadi, et al. "Effects of a Paleolithic Diet on Cardiovascular Disease Risk Factors: A Systematic Review and Meta-Analysis of Randomized Controlled Trials," *Advanced Nutrition* 10, no. 4 (April 2019): 634–46, DOI: 10.1093/advances/nmz007.

Manheimer, Eric W., Esther J. van Zuuren, Zbys Fedorowicz, and Hanno Pijl. "Paleo-lithic Nutrition for Metabolic Syndrome: Systematic Review and Meta-Analysis." *American Journal of Clinical Nutrition* 102, no. 4 (October 2015): 922–32. DOI: 10.3945 /ajcn.115.113613.

Otten, J., et al. "A Heterogeneous Response of Liver and Skeletal Muscle Fat to the Combination of a Paleolithic Diet and Exercise in Obese Individuals with Type 2 Diabetes: A Randomised Controlled Trial," *Diabetologia* 61, no. 7 (April 2018): 1548–59, DOI: 10.1007/s00125-018-4618-y.

Pastore, R. L., Judith T. Brooks, and John W. Carbone. "Paleolithic Nutrition Improves Plasma Lipid Concentrations of Hypercholesterolemic Adults to a Greater Extent Than Traditional Heart-Healthy Dietary Recommendations," *Nutrition Research* 35, no. 6 (June 2015): 474–79, DOI: 10.1016/j.nutres .2015.05.002.

Index

Acknowledgments

KINSEY JACKSON

This book is dedicated to the miracles in my life. To Jayne "Mila" Mardesich, you are a gift to those lucky enough to know you and living proof that a determined attitude is the most potent medicine of all. To my darling Milagro, the rainbow I've chased all my life, thank you for choosing me as your mama. I adore your fighter spirit and can't wait to watch you take this world by storm. Always remember that where there is love, there are miracles. And to my soul mate, Matthew, for always and forever.

SALLY JOHNSON

To my family: Thank you for eating my Paleo meals; they are always prepared with love. To my loving mother: Thank you for inspiring and initiating me into the world of nutrition. To my CrossFit community: Thank you for lighting the spark and always pushing me to the best version of myself. And to the ARC community: Here's to eating real food in a processed-food world!

About the Authors

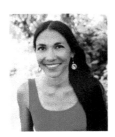

Kinsey Jackson, MS, CNS®, is a certified nutrition specialist clinician and certified functional medicine practitioner with a master of science in human nutrition. She specializes in the connection between diet and disease and has worked in the healthcare field for more than two decades. She is the author of four books, including *The Thyroid Reboot*. You can learn more about Kinsey at KinseyJackson.com.

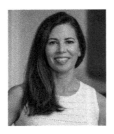

Sally Johnson, MA, RD, is a registered and licensed dietitian in Texas with a master's degree in applied physiology. She specializes in ancestral nutrition and is a certified functional medicine practitioner. Sally reversed her own health issues with functional nutrition and CrossFit. She now coaches clients on processed-food-addiction recovery. You can learn more at SallyJohnsonRD.com.

Printed in the USA
CPSIA information can be obtained
at www.ICGtesting.com
CBHW061309270624
10726CB00002B/5